Quick & Easy
LOW-CARB
RECIPES
for Beginners

Quarto.com

© 2023 Quarto Publishing Group USA Inc.
Text © 2002 Dana Carpender

First Published in 2023 by New Shoe Press, an imprint of The Quarto Group,
100 Cummings Center, Suite 265-D, Beverly, MA 01915, USA.
T (978) 282-9590 F (978) 283-2742

New Shoe Press titles are also available at discount for retail, wholesale, promotional, and bulk purchase. For details, contact the Special Sales Manager by email at specialsales@quarto.com or by mail at The Quarto Group, Attn: Special Sales Manager, 100 Cummings Center, Suite 265-D, Beverly, MA 01915, USA.

ISBN: 978-0-7603-8364-3
eISBN: 978-0-7603-8365-0

The content in this book was previously published in *500 Low-Carb Recipes* (Fair Winds Press 2003) by Dana Carpender.

Library of Congress Cataloging-in-Publication Data available

Cover Image: © Shutterstock

The information in this book is for educational purposes only. It is not intended to replace the advice of a physician or medical practitioner. Please see your health-care provider before beginning any new health program.

Quick & Easy
LOW-CARB
RECIPES
for Beginners

DANA CARPENDER

Low-Prep, No-Fuss Meals and Snacks for an Easy Low-Carb Lifestyle

NEW SHOE PRESS

Contents

Why Is There Such a Wide Range of Carb Counts in the Recipes in This Book?

If carbs are your problem, then they're going to be your problem tomorrow, and next week, and next year, and when you're old and gray. If you hope to keep your weight off, you cannot think in terms of going on a low-carb diet, losing your weight, and then going off your diet—you'll gain back every ounce, just as sure as you're born. You'll also go back to blood-sugar swings, energy crashes, and nagging, insatiable hunger, not to mention all the health risks of hyperinsulinemia. In short, you are in this for life.

So if you are to have any hope of doing this forever—and at this writing, I've been doing this for going on seven years—you're going to need to enjoy what you eat. You're going to need variety, flavor, color, and interest. You're going to need festive dishes, easy dishes, and comfort foods—a whole world of things to eat. You're going to need a cuisine.

Because of this, I have included everything from very low-carb dishes, suitable for folks in the early, very low-carb "induction" stage of their diet, to "splurge" dishes, which would probably make most of us gain weight if we ate them every day but which still have far fewer carbs than their "normal" counterparts.

There's another reason for the range of carb counts: Carbohydrate intol-erance comes in degrees, and different people can tolerate different daily carbohydrate intakes. Some of you, no doubt, need to stay in that 20-grams-a-day-or-less range, whereas many others—lucky souls—can have as much as 90 to 100 grams a day and stay slim. This cookbook is meant to serve you all.

Only you can know, through trial and error, how many grams of carbs you can eat in a day and still lose weight. It is up to you to pick and choose among the recipes in this book while keeping an eye on the carbohydrate counts provided. That way, you can put together menus that will please your palate and your family while staying below that critical carb level.

However, I do have this to say: Always, always, always the heart and soul of your low-carbohydrate diet should be meat, fish, poultry, eggs, healthy fats, and low-carb vegetables. This book will teach you a boggling number of ways to combine these things, and you should try them all. Don't just find one or two recipes that you like and make them over and over. Try at least one new recipe every week; that way, within a few months you'll have a whole new repertoire of familiar low-carb favorites!

You will, as I just mentioned, find recipes in this book for what are best considered low-carb treats. Do not take the presence of a recipe in this book to mean that it is something that you can eat every day, in unlimited quantities, and still lose weight. I can tell you from experience that even low-carb treats, if eaten frequently, will put weight on you. Recipes for breads, cookies, muffins, cakes, and the like are here to give you a satisfying, varied diet that you can live with for life, but they should not become the new staples of your diet. Do not try to make your low-carbohydrate diet resemble your former Standard American Diet. That's the diet that got you in trouble in the first place, remember?

One other thought: It is entirely possible to have a bad reaction to a food that has nothing to do with its carbohydrate count. Gluten, a protein from wheat that is essential for baking low-carb bread, causes bad reactions in a fair number of people. Soy products are problematic for many folks, as are nuts. Whey protein, used extensively in these recipes, con-tains lactose, which some people cannot tolerate. And surely you've heard of people who react badly to artificial sweeteners of one kind or another. I've also heard from diabetics who get bad blood-sugar spikes from eating even small quantities of onions or tomatoes.

Yet all of these foods are just fine for many, many low-carb dieters, and there is no way I can know which foods may cause a problem for which people. All I can tell you is to pay attention to your body. If you add a new food to your diet and you gain weight (and you're pretty certain it's not tied to something else, like your menstrual cycle or a new medication), or you find yourself unreasonably hungry, tired, or "off" despite having stayed within your body's carbohydrate tolerance, you may want to consider avoiding that food. One man's meat is another man's poison, and all that.

What's a "Usable Carb Count"?

Fiber is a carbohydrate and is, at least in American nutritional breakdowns, included in the total carbohydrate count. However, fiber is a form of carbohydrate made of molecules so big that you can neither digest nor absorb them. Therefore fiber, despite being a carbohydrate, will not push up your blood sugar and will not cause an insulin release. Even better, by slowing the absorption of the starches and sugars that occur with it, fiber actually lessens their bad influence. This is very likely the reason that high-fiber diets appear to be so much better for you than "American Normal."

These are the "usable" carbs, or the "effective carb count." These non-fiber grams of carbohydrates are what we count and limit. Not only does this approach allow us a much wider variety of foods, and especially lots more vegetables, but it actually encourages us to add fiber to things such as baked goods. I am very much a fan of this approach, and therefore I give the usable carbohydrate count for these recipes. However, you will also find the breakdown of the total carb count and the fiber count.

Using This Book

I can't tell you how to plan your menus. I don't know if you live alone or have a family, if you have hours to cook or are pressed for time every evening, or what foods are your favorites. I can, however, give you a few pointers on what you'll find here that may make your meal planning easier.

There are a lot of one-dish meals in this book—main dish salads, skillet suppers that include meat and vegetables both, and hearty soups that are a full meal in a bowl. If you have a carb-eating family, you can appease them by serving something on the side, such as whole wheat pitas split in half and toasted, along with garlic butter, brown rice, a baked potato, or some noodles. (Of course I don't recommend that you serve them something like canned biscuits, Tater Tots, or Minute Rice, but that shouldn't surprise you.)

When you're serving these one-dish meals, remember that most of your carbohydrate allowance for the meal is included in that main dish. Remember, it's the total usable carb count you have to keep an eye on. Complement simple meat dishes—such as roasted chicken, broiled steak, or pan-broiled pork chops—with the more carbohydrate-rich vegetable side dishes.

There's one other thing I hope this book teaches you to do, and that's break out of your old ways of looking at food.

Helpful General Hints

- If you're not losing weight, go back to counting every carb. Remember that snacks and beverages count, even if they're made from recipes in this book. A 6-gram muffin may be a lot better for you and your waistline than a convenience store muffin, but it's still 6 grams, and it counts! Likewise, don't lie to yourself about portion sizes. If you make your cookies really big, so that you only get two dozen instead of four dozen from a recipe, the carb count per cookie doubles, and don't you forget it.

- Beware of hidden carbohydrates. It's important to know that the government lets food manufacturers put "0 grams of carbohydrates" on the label if a food has less than 0.5 gram per serving, and "less than 1 gram of carbohydrate" if a food has between 0.5 gram and 0.9 gram. Even some diet sodas contain trace amounts of carbohydrates! These amounts aren't much, but they do add up if you eat enough of them. So if you're having trouble losing, count foods that say "0 grams" as 0.5 gram and foods that say "less than 1 gram" as 1 gram.

- Remember that some foods you may be thinking of as carb-free actually contain at least traces of carbohydrates. Eggs contain about 0.5 gram apiece, shrimp have 1 gram per 4-ounce portion, natural cheeses have about 1 gram per ounce, and heavy cream has about 0.5 gram per tablespoon. And coffee has more than 1 gram in a 10-ounce mug before you add cream and sweetener. (Tea, on the other hand, is carb-free.) If you're having trouble losing weight, get a food counter book and use it, even for foods you're sure you already know the carb counts of.

How Are the Carbohydrate Counts Calculated?

Most of these carbohydrate counts have been calculated using MasterCook software. This very useful program allows you to enter the ingredients of a recipe and the number of servings it makes, and it then spits out the nutritional breakdown for each serving. MasterCook does not include every low-carb specialty product, so these were looked up in food count books or on the product labels and added in by hand. Some figures were also derived from Corinne T. Netzer's *The Complete Book of Food Counts* and *The NutriBase Complete Book of Food Counts*. I have also used the FoodData Central, a hugely useful online reference.

The carb counts for these recipes are as accurate as we can make them. However, they are not, and cannot be, 100 percent accurate. MasterCook gets its nutritional information from the USDA Nutrient Database, and my experience is that the USDA's figures for carbohydrate content tend to run a bit higher than the food count books. This means that the carbo-hydrate counts in this book are, if anything, a tad high, which beats being too low!

Furthermore, every stalk of celery, every onion, every head of broccoli is going to have a slightly different level of carbohydrates in it, because it grew in a specific patch of soil, in specific weather, and with a particular kind of fertilizer. You may use a different brand of vanilla-flavored whey protein powder than I do. You may be a little more or a little less generous with how many bits of chopped green pepper you fit into a measuring cup. Don't sweat it. These counts are, as the old joke goes, close enough for government work. You can count on them as a guide to the carb content in your diet. And do you really want to get obsessed with getting every tenth of a gram written down?

In this spirit, you'll find that many of these recipes call for "1 large rib of celery," "half a green pepper," or "a clove of garlic." This is how most of us cook, after all. These things don't come in standard sizes, so they're analyzed for the average. Again: Don't sweat it! If you're really worried, use what seems to you a smallish stalk of celery, or green pepper, or clove of garlic, and you can count on your cumulative carb count being a hair lower than what is listed in the recipe.

Low-Carb Specialty Foods

Here's a taste of the variety of low-carb specialty products:

- **Breads and bagels.** These are often quite good, but keep an eye on the portion size listed on the label. I've seen low-carb bagels with a label claiming only 4 grams per serving, but discovered that a serving was only ⅓ of a bagel!

- **Tortillas.** Useful not only for eating with fajitas and burritos and for making quesadillas, but also in place of Chinese mu shu pancakes. Be aware that low-carb tortillas, although tasty, are not identical to either flour or corn tortillas in either flavor or texture.

- **Jams, jellies, and condiments.** These do contain the carbohydrates from whatever fruit or vegetable was used to make them, but not added sugars. Generally very good in quality, especially Jok'n Al brand, imported from New Zealand.

- **Pastas.** I have yet to find a brand of low-carb pasta that has really impressed me, but some of them are okay. I find that the texture of the pastas is off, so they cook up either too soft or too chewy. Still, the stuff sells like low-carb hotcakes, so somebody must really like it.

- **Cold cereals.** I've tried two low-carb cold cereals. One, called Keto Crisp, is quite similar to Rice Krispies in texture and flavor. This is now available in a chocolate flavor, as well. The other is called Nuttlettes, and it's very much like Grape Nuts. They're both good if you're fond of the cereals they imitate. Both of these "cereals" are made from soy, which some people think is a life-saving wonder food but others—including me—aren't sure is safe in large quantities. It's a moot point for me, since I just don't miss Rice Krispies or Grape Nuts enough to bother with these cereals. (Although Keto Crisp makes a mean cookie bar!) However, if you do miss cold cereal, these products are quite good, as well as low in carbohydrates and high in protein.

- **Protein chips.** These are okay, but not so wonderful that I've bothered to buy them often. Of the "regular" chips, these most closely resemble tortilla chips, but the texture is noticeably different. If you're mad for a bag of chips, these are worth a try. But for me, I'd rather have pumpkin seeds.

- **Protein meal replacement shakes.** Mostly quite good, and certainly useful for folks who can't face cooked food first thing in the morning. They're available in a wide range of flavors.

- **Protein bars.** These seem to be everywhere these days. They range from pretty darned good to absolutely wretched, sometimes within the same brand. You'll have to try a few brands and flavors to see which ones you like. Be aware that there is a lot of controversy about low-carb protein bars. Virtually all of them contain glycerine, to make them moist and chewy. The controversy is over whether or not glycerine acts like a carbohydrate in some ways in the body. Many people find that these bars knock them out of ketosis, whereas others don't have a problem. So I'll say it again: Pay attention to your body!

- **Hot cereal.** There is one low-carb hot cereal on the market at this writing: Flax-O-Meal. I haven't tried it, but by all reports it is very good.

- **Cookies and brownies.** These are getting better every day, and many are quite good already. I've had low-carb brownies that were superb, and some very nice oatmeal cookies, as well. See "About Polyols," on page 10.

- **Muffins.** Although some of these are quite good, others are not so brilliant, and often the same brand varies widely depending on which flavor you choose. You'll just have to try them and see which you like.

- **Other sweet low-carb baked goods.** I've tried commercially made low-carb cheesecake and cake rolls. The cheesecake was pretty good, but I can make better for far less money. I didn't like the cake rolls at all because I found them overwhelmingly sweet. But I know that they sell quite well, so somebody must like them.

- **Chocolate bars and other chocolate candy.** These, my friend, are generally superb. The best of the low-carb chocolate candies, including Carbolite, Pure De-Lite, Ross, Darrell Lea, and Low Carb Chef, are indistinguishable from their sugar-laden counterparts. You can get low-carb chocolate in both milk and dark. There are peanut butter cups, crispy bars, turtles, you name it. I haven't had a really bad sugar-free chocolate yet. See "About Polyols," below.

- **Other sugar-free candy.** You can, if you look, find sugar-free taffies, hard candies, marshmallows, jelly beans, and other sweet treats. Again, the quality of these tends to be excellent. See "About Polyols," below.

About Polyols

Polyols, also known as sugar alcohols, are widely used in sugar-free candies and cookies. There are a variety of polyols, and their names all end with "ol"—lactitol, maltitol, mannitol, sorbitol, xylitol, and the like. Polyols are, indeed, carbohydrates, but they are carbohydrates that are made up of molecules that are too big for humans to digest or absorb easily. As a result, polyols don't create much, if any, rise in blood sugar, nor do they create much of an insulin release.

Polyols are used in commercial sugar-free sweets because, unlike Splenda and other artificial sweeteners, they will give all of the textures that can be achieved with sugar. Polyols can be used to make crunchy toffee, chewy jelly beans, slick hard candies, chewy brownies, and creamy chocolate, just as sugar can. Yet they are far, far easier on your carbohydrate metabolism, and on your teeth, as well.

However, there are one or two problems with polyols. First of all, there is some feeling that different people have different abilities to digest and absorb these very long chain carbohydrates, which means that for some people, polyols may cause more of a derangement of blood sugar than they do for others. Once again, my only advice is to pay attention to your body.

The other problem with polyols is one that is inherent in all indigestible, unabsorbable carbohydrates: They can cause gas and diarrhea. Unabsorbed carbs ferment in your gut, creating intestinal gas as a result. It's the exact same thing that happens when people eat beans. I find that even half of a low-carb chocolate bar is enough to cause me social embarrassment several hours later. And I know of a case where eating a dozen and a half sugar-free taffies before bed caused the hapless consumer 45 minutes of serious gut-cramping intestinal distress at 4 a.m.

Don't think, by the way, that you can get around these effects of polyol consumption by taking Beano. This will work, but it will work by making the carbohydrates digestible and absorbable. This means that any low-carb advantage is gone. I know folks who have gained weight this way.

What we have here, then, is a sweetener that enforces moderation. Personally, I think this is a wonderful thing.

How much you can eat in the way of polyol-sweetened products without getting into digestive trouble will vary with each food's polyol content. For instance, sugar-free taffy is almost solid polyols, just as its sugary counterpart is virtually all sugar. Sugar-free chocolate, on the other hand, has much of its bulk made up of the chocolate. The bottom line is, I wouldn't eat sugar-free candies at all if you have an important meeting or a hot date a few hours later, or if you'll be getting on an airplane. (Altitude can make gas swell very uncomfortably in your gut.) If you can afford some gaseousness, for lack of a better word, I'd stick to no more than one chocolate bar or three or four taffies or caramels in a day.

One more good thing to know about polyols: It's not just candies that are labeled "low carbohydrate" that are made with these sweeteners. Many well-known candy companies, such as Fannie May and Fannie Farmer, make sugar-free chocolates, and virtually all of them use polyols. The only difference is that they count the carbohydrate grams in the polyols in their nutrition counts, even though the polyols are not, for the most part, absorbed. If you see a candy labeled "sugar free" that you're interested in, don't ask for the carb count, ask what it's sweetened with. If it's sweetened with something ending in "ol," chances are that it's okay for you. But once again, do pay attention to your body's reaction.

Where to Find Low-Carbohydrate Specialty Products

The availability of low-carbohydrate specialty products varies a great deal. Health food stores are good places to start your search, but even though some will carry these products, others still are caught up in low-fat, whole grain mania, and therefore shun them. Some carry things like fiber crackers and protein powder, but refuse to carry anything artificial-ly sweetened because they pride themselves on carrying "natural" products only. Still, you'll want to find a good health food store to use as a source of many ingredients called for in this book, especially those for low-carb baking, so you may as well go poke around any health food stores in your area and see what you can find.

Little specialty groceries often carry low-carbohydrate products as a way to attract new and repeat business. In my town, Sahara Mart, a store that has long specialized in Middle Eastern foods, has become the best source for low-carb specialty products, as well. If a store carries a broad line of products specifically for low-carb dieters, they'll generally advertise it with signs in the windows, so keep your eyes open.

If you can't find a local source for such things as sugar-free chocolate, low-carb pasta, or whatever else you want, your best bet is to go online. Hit your favorite search engine, and search for "low-carbohydrate products," "sugar-free candy," or whatever it is you're looking for. There are a whole lot of low-carb "e-tailers" out there; find the ones with the products and prices you want. If you don't care to use your credit card online, most of them have toll-free order numbers you can call, and others have the ability to take checks online, as well as credit cards. A few companies I've done business with happily are Carb Smart, Low Carb Grocery, and Synergy Diet, but there are tons of them out there if you take the time to look.

On the Importance of Reading Labels

Do yourself a favor and get in the habit of reading the label on every food product, and I do mean every food product, that has one. I have learned from long, hard, repetitive experience that food manufacturers can, will, and do put sugar, corn syrup, corn starch, and other nutritionally empty, carb-laden garbage into every conceivable food product. I have found sugar in everything from salsa to canned clams, for heaven's sake! (Who it was who thought that the clams needed sugaring, I'd love to know.) You will shave untold thousands of grams of carbs off your intake in the course of a year by simply looking for the product that has no added junk.

There are also a good many classes of food products out there to which sugar is virtually always added; the cured meats come to mind. There is almost always sugar in sausage, ham, bacon, hot dogs, liverwurst, and the like. You will look in vain for sugarless varieties of these products, which is one good reason why you should primarily eat fresh meats, instead.

CHAPTER 1

Ingredients You Need to Know About

This is by no means an exhaustive rundown of every single ingredient used in this book; these are just the ones I thought you might have questions about. I've grouped them by use, and within those groupings they're alphabetized, so if you have a question about something used in a recipe, flip back here and read up on whatever you're curious about.

Fats and Oils

Bland Oils

Sometimes you want a bland oil in a recipe, something that adds little or no flavor of its own. In that case, I recommend peanut, sunflower, or canola oil. These are the oils I mean when I simply specify "oil" in a recipe. Avoid highly polyunsaturated oils such as safflower; they deteri-orate quickly both from heat and from contact with oxygen, and they've been associated with an increased risk of cancer.

Butter

When a recipe says butter, use butter, will you? Margarine is nasty, unhealthy stuff, full of hydrogenated oils, trans fats, and artificial everything. It's terrible for you. So use the real thing. If real butter strains your budget, watch for sales and stock up; butter freezes beautifully.

Coconut Oil

Coconut oil makes an excellent substitute for hydrogenated vegetable shortening (Crisco and the like), which you should shun. Surprisingly, it has no coconut flavor or aroma; you can use it for sautéing or in baking without adding any "off" flavor to your recipes.

Olive Oil

It surely will come as no surprise to you that olive oil is a healthy fat, but you may not know that there are various kinds. Extra-virgin olive oil is the first pressing. It is deep green, with a full, fruity flavor, and it makes all the difference in salad dressings.

For sautéing and other general uses, I use a grade of olive oil known as "pomace." Pomace is far cheaper than extra-virgin olive oil, and it has a milder flavor. These gallon cans are worth looking for because they're the cheapest way to buy the stuff. If you can't find gallon cans of pomace, feel free to buy whatever cheaper, milder-flavored type of olive oil is available at your grocery store.

Flour Substitutes

As you are no doubt aware, flour is out, for the most part, in low-carb cooking. Flour serves a few different purposes in cooking, from making up the bulk of most baked goods and creating stretchiness in bread dough to thickening sauces and "binding" casseroles. In low-carb cooking, we use different ingredients for these various purposes. Here's a rundown of flour substitutes you'll want to have on hand for low-carb cooking and baking:

Brans

Because fiber is a carbohydrate that we neither digest nor absorb, brans of one kind or another are very useful for bulking up (no pun intended!) low-carb baked goods. I use different kinds in different recipes. You'll want to have at least wheat bran and oat bran on hand; both of these are widely available. If you can also find rice bran, it's worth picking up, especially if you have high cholesterol. Of all the kinds of bran tested, rice bran was most powerful for lowering high blood cholesterol.

Ground Almonds and Hazelnuts

Finely ground almonds and hazelnuts are wonderful for replacing some or all of the flour in many recipes, especially cakes and cookies. If you can purchase almond meal and hazelnut meal locally, these should work fine in the recipes in this book. If you can't (I don't have a local source for these), simply grind nuts in your food processor, using the S blade. The nuts are not the texture of flour when ground, but more the consistency of coarsely ground cornmeal. Whenever a recipe in this book calls for ground almonds or hazelnuts, this is what I used.

It's good to know that these nuts actually expand a little during grinding. This surprised me because I thought they'd compress a bit. Figure that between ⅔ and ¾ of a cup of either of these nuts will become 1 cup when ground.

Guar and Xanthan Gums

Guar and xanthan are both flavorless white powders; their value to us is as low-carb thickeners. Technically speaking, these are carbs, but they're all fiber, nothing but, so don't worry about using them.

You'll find guar or xanthan used in small quantities in a lot of these recipes. Don't go dramatically increasing the quantity of guar or xanthan to get a thicker product, because in large quantities they make things gummy, and the texture is not terribly pleasant. But in these tiny quantities they add oomph to sauces and soups without using flour. You can always leave the guar or xanthan out if you can't find it; you'll just get a somewhat thinner result.

You'll notice that I always tell you to put the guar or xanthan through the blender with whatever liquid it is that you're using. This is because it is very difficult to simply whisk guar into a sauce and not get little gummy lumps in your finished sauce or soup, and the blender is the best way to thoroughly combine your ingredients.

If you don't own or don't want to use a blender, there is one possible alternative: Put your guar or xanthan in a salt shaker, and sprinkle it, bit by bit, over your sauce, stirring madly all the while with a whisk. The problem here, of course, is there's no way to know exactly how much you're using, so you'll just have to stop when your dish reaches the degree of thickness you like. Still, this can be a useful trick.

Low-Carbohydrate Bake Mix

There are several brands of low-carbohydrate bake mix on the market. These are generally a combination of some form of powdery protein and fiber, such as soy, whey, and sometimes oat, plus baking powder, and sometimes salt. These mixes are the low-carb world's equivalent of Bisquick, although low-carb bake mixes differ from Bisquick in that they do not have shortening added. You will need to add butter, oil, or some other form of fat when using them to make pancakes, waffles, biscuits, and such. I mostly use low-carb bake mix in lesser quantities, for "flouring" chicken before baking or frying, or replacing flour as a "binder" in a casserole.

Oat Flour

One or two recipes in this book call for oat flour. Because of its high fiber content, oat flour has a lower usable carb count than most other flours. Even so, it must be used in very small quantities. Oat flour is available at health food stores. In a pinch, you can grind up oatmeal in your blender or food processor.

Psyllium Husks

This is another fiber product. It's the same form of fiber that is used in Metamucil and similar products. Because psyllium has little flavor of its own, it makes a useful high-fiber "filler" in some low-carb bread recipes. Look for plain psyllium husks at your health food store. Mine carries them in bulk, quite cheaply, but if yours doesn't, look for them among the laxatives and "colon health" products.

Rice Protein Powder

For savory recipes such as entrees, you need a protein powder that isn't sweet, and preferably one that has no flavor at all. There are a number of these on the market, and some are blander than others. I tried several kinds, and I've found that rice protein powder is the one I like best. I buy Nutribiotics brand, which has 1 gram of carbohydrates per tablespoon, but any unflavored rice protein powder with a similar carb count should work fine. For that matter, I see no reason not to experiment with other unflavored protein powders, if you like.

Rolled Oats

Also known as old-fashioned oatmeal, rolled oats are oat grains that have been squashed flat. These are available in every grocery store in the Western Hemisphere. Do not substitute instant or quick-cooking oatmeal.

Soy Powder, Soy Flour, and Soy Protein Isolate

Some of my recipes call for soy powder. None call for soy flour, although a few recipes from other folks do. If you use soy flour in a recipe that calls for soy powder, you won't get the results I got. You also won't get the right results with soy protein powder, also known as soy protein isolate. What is the difference? Soy protein isolate is a protein that has been extracted from soybeans and concentrated into a protein powder. Soy flour is made from raw soybeans that have simply been ground up into flour, and it has a strong bean flavor. Soy powder, also known as soy milk powder, is made from whole soybeans, like soy flour, but the beans are cooked before they're ground up. For some reason I don't pretend to understand, this gets rid of the strong flavor and makes soy powder taste quite mild.

You should be aware that despite the tremendous marketing buildup soy has enjoyed for the past several years, there are some problems emerging. Soy is well known to interfere with thyroid function, which is the last thing you need if you're trying to lose weight. It also can interfere with mineral absorption. It is also less certain, but still possible, that regular consumption of soy causes brain deterioration and genital defects in boy babies born to mothers with soy-heavy diets. For these reasons, although I do not shun soy entirely, I use other options when possible.

Vital Wheat Gluten

Gluten is a grain protein. It's the gluten in flour that makes bread dough stretchy so that it will trap the gas released by the yeast, letting your bread rise. We are not, of course, going to use regular, all-purpose flour, with its high carbohydrate content. Fortunately, it is possible to buy concentrated wheat gluten. This high-protein, low-starch flour is absolutely essential to making low-carbohydrate yeast breads.

To make sure you're getting the right product, you'll simply have to read the label. The product you want,

regardless of what the packager calls it, will have between 75 and 80 percent protein, or about 24 grams in ¼ cup. It will also have a very low carbohydrate count, somewhere in the neighborhood of 6 grams of carbohydrates in that same ¼ cup. If your health food store has a bulk bin labeled "high-gluten flour" or "gluten flour" but there's no nutrition label attached, ask to see the bulk food manager and request the information off of the sack the flour came in. If the label on the bin says "vital wheat gluten" or "pure gluten flour," you can probably trust it.

At this writing, the most widely distributed brand of vital wheat gluten in the United States is Bob's Red Mill.

Wheat Germ

The germ is the part of the wheat kernel that would have become the plant if the grain had sprouted. It is the most nutritious, highest protein part of the wheat kernel, and is much lower in carbohydrates than the starchy part that becomes white flour. A few recipes in this book call for raw wheat germ, which is available at health food stores. Raw wheat germ should be refrigerated, as it goes rancid pretty easily. If your health food store doesn't keep the raw wheat germ in the cooler, I'd look for another health food store.

Whey Protein Powder

Whey is the liquid part of milk. If you've ever seen yogurt that has separated, the clearish liquid on top is the whey. Whey protein is of extremely good quality, and the protein powder made from it is tops in both flavor and nutritional value. For any sweet recipe, the vanilla-flavored whey protein powder is best, and it's readily available in health food stores. Keep in mind that protein powders vary in their carbohydrate counts, so look for the one with the fewest carbohydrates. Also beware of sugar-sweetened protein powders, which can be higher in carbs. The one I use is sweetened with stevia and has a little less than 1 gram of carbohydrates per tablespoon.

Natural whey protein powder is just like vanilla-flavored whey protein powder, except that it has not been flavored or sweetened. Its flavor is bland, so it is used in recipes where a sweet flavor is not desirable. Natural whey protein powder is called for in some of the recipes that other folks have donated to this book; I generally use rice protein powder when a bland protein powder is called for.

Liquids

Broths

Canned or boxed chicken and beef broths are very handy items to keep around, and it's certainly quicker to make dinner with these than it would be if you had to make your own from scratch. However, the quality of most of the canned broth you'll find at your local grocery store is appallingly bad. The chicken broth has all sorts of chemicals in it and often sugar, as well. The "beef" broth is worse, frequently containing no beef whatsoever. I refuse to use these products, and you should, too.

Decent packaged broth won't cost you a whole lot more than the stuff that is made of salt and chemicals. If you watch for sales, you can often get it as cheaply as the bad stuff; stock up on it then.

One last note: You will also find canned vegetable broth, particularly at health food stores. This is tasty, but it runs much higher in carbohydrates than the chicken and beef broths. I'd avoid it.

Vinegar

Various recipes in this book call for wine vinegar, cider vinegar, sherry vinegar, rice vinegar, tarragon vinegar, white vinegar, balsamic vinegar, and even raspberry vinegar, for which you'll find a recipe. If you've always thought that vinegar was just vinegar, think again! Each of these vinegars has a distinct flavor all its own, and if you substitute one for the other, you'll change the whole character of the recipe. Add just one splash of cider vinegar to your Asian Chicken Salad (see page 102), and you've traded your Chinese accent for an American twang. Vinegar is such a great way to give bright flavors to foods while adding very few carbs that I keep all of these varieties on hand. This is easy to do, because vinegar keeps for a very long time.

As with everything else, read the labels on your vinegar. I've seen cider vinegar that has 0 grams of carbohydrates per ounce and I've seen cider vinegar that has 4 grams of carbohydrates per ounce—a huge difference. Beware, also, of apple cider–flavored vinegar, which is white vinegar with artificial flavors added. I bought this once by mistake. (You'd think someone who constantly reminds others to read labels would be beyond such errors, wouldn't you?)

Wine

There are several recipes in this cookbook calling for either dry red or dry white wine. I find the inexpensive box wines, which come in a mylar bag inside a cardboard box, very convenient to keep on hand for cooking. The simple reason for this is that they don't go bad because the contents are never exposed to air. These are not fabulous vintage wines, but they're fine for our modest purposes, and they certainly are handy. I generally have both Burgundy and Chablis wine-in-a-box on hand. Be wary of any wine with "added flavors." Too often, one of those flavors will be sugar. Buy wine with a recognizable name, such as Burgundy, Rhine, Chablis, Cabernet, and the like, rather than stuff like "Chillable Red," and you'll get better results.

Nuts, Seeds, and Nut Butters

Nuts and Seeds

Low in carbohydrates and high in healthy fats, protein, and minerals, nuts and seeds are great foods for us. Not only are they delicious for snacking or for adding crunch to salads and stir-fries, but when ground, they can replace some of the flour in low-carb baked goods. In particular, you'll find quite a few recipes in this book calling for ground almonds, ground hazelnuts, and ground sunflower seeds. Since these ingredients can be pricey, you'll want to shop around. In particular, health food stores often carry nuts and seeds in bulk at better prices than you'll find at the grocery store. I have also found that specialty ethnic groceries often have good prices on nuts. I get my best deal on almonds at my wonderful Middle Eastern grocery, Sahara Mart.

By the way, along with pumpkin and sunflower seeds, you can buy sesame seeds in bulk at health food stores for a fraction of what they'll cost you in a little shaker jar at the grocery store. Buy them "unhulled" and you'll get both more fiber and more calcium. You can also get unsweetened coconut flakes at health food stores.

Flaxseed comes from the same plant that gives us the fabric linen, and it is turning out to be one of the most nutritious seeds there is. Along with good-quality protein, flaxseeds have tons of soluble, cholesterol-reducing fiber and are a rich source of eicosapentaenoic acid (EPA), the same fats that make fish so heart-healthy.

Most of the recipes in this book that use flaxseed call for it to be ground up into a coarse meal. You can buy pre-ground flaxseed meal (Bob's Red Mill sells it, among others), but I much prefer to grind my own. The simple reason for this is that the fats in flaxseeds are very stable so long as the seeds are whole, but they go rancid pretty quickly after the seed coat is broken.

Grinding flaxseed is very easy if you have a food processor. Simply put the seeds in your food processor with the S blade in place, turn on the machine, and forget about it for about 5 minutes. (Yes, it takes that long!) You can then add your flaxseed meal to whatever it is you're cooking.

If you don't have a food processor, you'll just have to buy flaxseed meal pre-ground. If you do, keep it in an airtight container, refrigerate or freeze it, and use it up as quickly as you can.

Nut Butters

The only peanut butter called for in this cookbook is "natural" peanut butter, the kind made from ground, roasted peanuts; peanut oil; salt; and nothing else. Most big grocery stores now carry natural peanut butter; it's the stuff with the layer of oil on top. The oil in standard peanut butter has been hydrogenated to keep it from separating out (that's what gives big name-brand peanut butters that extremely smooth, plastic consistency) and it's hard to think of anything worse for you than hydrogenated vegetable oil—except for sugar, of course, which is also added to standard peanut butter. Stick to the natural stuff.

Grocery stores carry not only natural peanut butter but also almond butter, sunflower butter, and sesame butter, generally called "tahini." All of these are useful for low-carbers. Keep all natural nut butters in the refrigerator unless you're going to eat them up within a week or two.

Seasonings

Bouillon or Broth Concentrates

Bouillon or broth concentrate comes in cubes, crystals, or liquids. It is generally full of salt and chemicals, and it doesn't taste notably like the animal it supposedly came from. It definitely does not make a suitable substitute for good-quality broth if you're making a pot of soup. However, these products can be useful for adding a little kick of flavor here and there, more as seasonings than as soups, and for this, I keep them on hand. I generally use chicken bouillon crystals because I find them easier to use than cubes. I also keep liquid beef broth concentrate on hand. I chose this because, unlike the cubes or crystals it actually has a bit of beef in it. I use Wyler's, but see no reason why any comparable product wouldn't work fine. If you can get the British product Bovril, it might even be better!

Fresh Ginger

Many recipes in this book call for fresh ginger, sometimes called gingerroot. Fresh ginger is an essential ingredient in Asian cooking, and dried, powdered ginger is not a substitute. Fortunately, fresh ginger freezes beautifully; just drop your whole gingerroot (called a "hand" of ginger) into a zipper-lock freezer bag, and toss it in the freezer. When the time comes to use it, pull it out, peel enough of the end for your immediate purposes, and grate it. (It will grate just fine while still frozen.) Throw the remaining root back in the bag, and toss it back on the freezer.

Garlic

Garlic is a borderline vegetable. It's fairly high in carbohydrates, but it's very, very good for you. Surely you've heard all about garlic's nutritional prowess by now. Garlic also, of course, is an essential flavoring ingredient in many recipes. However, remember that there is an estimated 1 gram of carbohydrates per clove, so go easy. A "clove," by the way, is one of those little individual bits you get in a whole garlic bulb. If you read "clove" and use a whole bulb (also called a "head") of garlic, you'll get lots more carbs—and a lot stronger garlic flavor—than you expected.

I only use fresh garlic, except for in the occasional recipe that calls for a sprinkle-on seasoning blend. Nothing else tastes like the real thing. To my taste buds, even the jarred, chopped garlic in oil doesn't taste like fresh garlic. And we won't even talk about garlic powder. You may use jarred garlic if you like; ½ teaspoon should equal about 1 clove of fresh garlic. If you choose to use powdered garlic, well, I can't stop you, but I'm afraid I can't promise the recipes will taste the same, either. Figure that ¼ teaspoon of garlic powder is roughly equivalent to 1 clove of fresh garlic.

Vege-Sal

If you've read my newsletter, Lowcarbezine!, you know that I'm a big fan of Vege-Sal. What is Vege-Sal? It's a salt that's been seasoned, but don't think "seasoned salt." Vege-Sal is much milder than traditional seasoned salt. It's simply salt that's been blended with some dried, powdered veg-etables. The flavor is quite subtle, but I think it improves all sorts of things. I've given you the choice between using regular salt or Vege-Sal in a wide variety of recipes. Don't worry, they'll come out fine with plain old salt, but I do think Vege-Sal adds a little something extra. Vege-Sal is also excellent sprinkled over chops and steaks in place of regular salt. Vege-Sal is made by Modern Products and is widely available.

Sweeteners

Blackstrap Molasses

What the heck is molasses doing in a low-carb cookbook? It's practically all carbohydrates, after all. Well, yes, but I've found that combining Splenda (see below) with a very small amount of molasses gives a good brown-sugar flavor to all sorts of recipes. Always use the darkest molasses you can find; the darker it is, the stronger the flavor and the lower the carb count. That's why I specify blackstrap—the darkest, strongest molasses there is. It's nice to know that blackstrap is also where all the minerals they take out of sugar end up, so it may be full of carbs, but at least it's not a nutritional wasteland. Still, I only use small amounts.

Most health food stores carry blackstrap molasses, but if you can't find it, always buy the darkest molasses available, keeping in mind that most grocery store brands come in both light and dark varieties.

Why not use some of the artificial brown sugar–flavored sweeteners out there? Because I've tried them, and I haven't tasted even one I would be willing to buy again. Ick.

Splenda

Splenda is the latest artificial sweetener to hit the market, and it blows all of the competition clear out of the water! Feed nondieting friends and family Splenda-sweetened desserts, and they will never know that you didn't use sugar. It tastes that good.

Splenda has some other advantages. The table sweetener has been bulked so that it measures just like sugar, spoon-for-spoon and cup-for-cup. This makes adapting recipes much easier. Also, Splenda stands up to heat, unlike aspartame, which means you can use it for baked goods and other things that are heated for a while.

However, Splenda is not completely carb-free. Because of the maltodextrin used to bulk it, Splenda has about 0.5 gram of carbohydrates per teaspoon, or about ⅛ of the carbohydrates of sugar. So count half a gram per teaspoon, 1½ grams per tablespoon, and 24 grams per cup. At this writing, McNeil, the company that makes Splenda, has no plans to release liquid Splenda in the United States, but I am hoping that they will change their minds. The liquid, available in some foreign countries, is carb-free. So while it will take a little more finesse to figure out quantities, it will also allow me to slash the carb counts of all sorts of recipes still further! Stay tuned.

Stevia/FOS Blend

Stevia is short for Stevia rebaudiana, a South American shrub with very sweet leaves. Stevia extract, a white powder from stevia leaves, is growing in popularity with people who don't care to eat sugar but who are nervous about artificial sweeteners.

However, stevia extract has a couple of faults: First, it's so extremely sweet that it's hard to know just how much to use in any given recipe. Second, it often has a bitter taste as well as a sweet one. This is why some smart food packagers have started blending stevia with fructooligosaccharide, also known as FOS. FOS is a sugar, but it's a sugar with a molecule so large that humans can neither digest nor absorb it, so it doesn't raise blood sugar or cause an insulin release. FOS has a nice, mild sweetness to it; indeed, it's only half as sweet as table sugar. This makes it the perfect partner for the too-sweet stevia.

This stevia/FOS blend is called for in just a few recipes in this book. It is available in many health food stores, both in packets and in shaker jars. The brand I use is called SteviaPlus, and it's from a company called Sweet Leaf, but any stevia/FOS blend should do for the recipes that call for it.

My favorite use for this stevia/FOS blend, by the way, is to sweeten my yogurt. I think it tastes quite good, and FOS actually helps the good bacteria take hold in your gut, improving your health.

CHAPTER 2

Hors D'oeuvres, Snacks, and Party Nibbles

Unlike most snack and party foods, the recipes in this chapter are actually nutritious and filling. This means two things: One, that if you serve one or two of these items before dinner, you may want to cut back a bit on quantities at the meal itself, and two, that you can actually use many of these recipes as light meals in and of themselves. This is a particularly nice idea for family movie night—just put out a big tray of cut up vegetables and dip, some wings, and a bowl of nut mix, and call it supper.

Hot Wings

If you want to simplify this recipe, use store-bought Buffalo Wing sauce instead of the mixture of dry spices. Most wing sauces don't have any sugar in them and are quite low in carbs.

1 teaspoon cayenne pepper

2 teaspoons dried oregano

1 teaspoon curry powder

2 teaspoons paprika

2 teaspoons dried thyme

2 pounds chicken wings, cut into drumettes

—

Yield: About 24 pieces, each with a trace of carbohydrates, a trace of fiber, and 4 grams of protein.

Preheat the oven to 375°F.

Combine the pepper, oregano, curry, paprika, and thyme well in a bowl.

Arrange the wings in a shallow baking pan, and sprinkle the mixture evenly over them, turning to coat both sides.

Roast for 45 to 50 minutes, or until crisp. Serve with the traditional accompaniments of ranch or blue cheese dressing and celery sticks, if desired.

Paprika Wings

20 chicken wing drumsticks

3 tablespoons olive oil

2 cloves garlic, crushed

Salt

Pepper

Paprika

—

Yield: 20 pieces, each with a trace of carbohydrates, a trace of fiber, and 4 grams of protein.

Preheat the oven to 350°F.

Arrange the wings in a baking pan so that they are not touching.

Combine the oil and garlic, and spoon the mixture over the wings. Make sure you get a little of the crushed garlic on each piece.

Sprinkle the wings with salt and pepper to taste, and then with enough paprika to make them reddish all over.

Roast for 15 to 20 minutes, then turn them over and sprinkle the other side with salt, pepper, and paprika.

Roast for another 45 minutes to 1 hour, turning every 15 to 20 minutes.

STUFFED EGGS

Don't save these recipes for parties: If you're a low-carb eater, a refrigerator full of stuffed eggs is a beautiful thing. Here are six varieties. Feel free to double or triple any of these recipes— you know they'll disappear.

Classic Deviled Eggs

These are everybody's potluck supper favorite.

6 hard-boiled eggs

5 tablespoons mayonnaise

2 teaspoons spicy brown or Dijon mustard

¼ teaspoon salt or Vege-Sal

Paprika

—

Yield: 12 halves, each with a trace of carbohydrates, a trace of fiber, and 3 grams of protein.

Slice the eggs in half, and carefully remove the yolks into a mixing bowl.

Mash the yolks with a fork. Stir in the mayonnaise, mustard, and salt, and mix until creamy.

Spoon the mixture back into the hollows in the egg whites. Sprinkle with a little paprika for color.

Onion Eggs

6 hard-boiled eggs

5 tablespoons mayonnaise

1 teaspoon spicy brown or Dijon mustard

2½ teaspoons very finely minced sweet red onion

5 drops Tabasco

¼ teaspoon salt or Vege-Sal

—

Yield: 12 halves, each with a trace of carbohydrates, a trace of fiber, and 3 grams of protein.

Slice the eggs in half, and carefully remove the yolks into a mixing bowl.

Mash the yolks with a fork. Stir in the mayonnaise, mustard, onion, Tabasco, and salt, and mix until creamy.

Spoon the mixture back into the hollows in the egg whites.

Artichoke Parmesan Dip

Serve this party favorite with pepper strips, cucumber rounds, celery sticks, or low-carb fiber crackers.

1 can (13½ ounces) artichoke hearts

1 cup mayonnaise

1 cup grated Parmesan cheese

1 clove garlic, crushed, or 1 teaspoon of jarred, chopped garlic

Paprika

—

Yield: 4 servings, each with 3 grams of carbohydrates and 1 gram of fiber, for a total of 2 grams of usable carbs and 10 grams of protein.

Preheat the oven to 325°F.

Drain and chop the artichoke hearts.

Mix the artichoke hearts with the mayonnaise, cheese, and garlic, combining well.

Put the mixture in a small, oven-proof casserole, sprinkle a little paprika on top, and bake for 45 minutes.

Spinach Artichoke Dip

This is a great, equally yummy version of the previous recipe, but keep in mind that it does make twice as much dip.

1 can (13½ ounces) artichoke hearts

1 package frozen chopped spinach (10 ounces), thawed

2 cups mayonnaise

2 cups grated Parmesan cheese

2 cloves garlic, crushed, or 2 teaspoons jarred, chopped garlic

Paprika

—

Yield: 8 servings, each with 4 grams of carbohydrates and 2 grams of fiber, for a total of 2 grams of usable carbs and 10 grams of protein.

Drain and chop the artichoke hearts.

Combine the spinach, mayonnaise, cheese, and garlic in a large casserole (a 6-cup dish is about right). Sprinkle with paprika.

Bake at 325°F for 50 to 60 minutes.

Guacamole

This is a very simple guacamole recipe, without sour cream or mayonnaise, that lets the taste of the avocados shine through.

4 ripe black avocados

2 tablespoons minced sweet red onion

3 tablespoons lime juice

3 cloves garlic, crushed

¼ teaspoon Tabasco

Salt or Vege-Sal to taste

—

Yield: 6 generous servings, each with 11 grams of carbohydrates and 3 grams of fiber, for a total of 8 grams of usable carbs and 3 grams of protein.

Halve the avocados, and scoop the flesh into a mixing bowl. Mash coarsely with a fork.

Mix in the onion, lime juice, garlic, Tabasco, and salt, stirring to blend well and mashing to the desired consistency.

WARNING

This recipe contains lots of healthy fats and almost three times the potassium found in a banana.

Dill Dip

This easy dip tastes wonderful with all sorts of raw vegetables; try serving it with celery, peppers, cucumber, broccoli, or whatever else you have on hand.

1 pint sour cream

¼ small onion

1 heaping tablespoon dry dill weed

½ teaspoon salt or Vege-Sal

—

Yield: 1 pint, containing 25 grams of carbohydrates and 1 gram of fiber, for a total of 24 grams of usable carbs and 16 grams of protein in the batch. (This is easily enough for 10 to 12 people, so no one's going to get more than a few grams of carbs.)

Put the sour cream, onion, dill weed, and salt in a food processor, and process until the onion disappears. (If you don't have a food processor, mince the onion very fine and just stir everything together.)

You can serve this right away, but it tastes even better if you let it chill for a few hours.

Clam Dip

With some celery sticks and pepper strips for scooping, this would make a good lunch. Of course you can serve it at parties, too, with celery, green pepper, cucumber rounds, or fiber crackers for you and crackers or chips for the non low-carbers.

2 packages (8 ounces each) cream cheese, softened

½ cup mayonnaise

2 to 3 teaspoons Worcestershire sauce

1 tablespoon Dijon mustard

8 to 10 scallions, including the crisp part of the green shoot, minced

2 cans (6½ ounces each) minced clams, drained

Salt or Vege-Sal

Pepper

—

Yield: 12 servings, each with just under 4 grams of carbohydrates, a trace of fiber, and 10 grams of protein.

Combine all the ingredients well, and chill. A food processor or blender works well for this, or if you prefer to leave chunks of clam, you could use an electric mixer.

Smoked Gouda Veggie Dip

Great with celery, peppers, or any favorite raw veggie. Combine your ingredients with a mixer, not a food processor, so you have actual little bits of Gouda in the dip.

1 package (8 ounces) cream cheese, softened

⅔ cup mayonnaise

1 cup shredded smoked Gouda

6 scallions, including the crisp part of the green shoot, sliced

2 tablespoons grated Parmesan cheese

½ teaspoon pepper

—

Yield: at least 8 servings, each with 2 grams of carbohydrates, a trace of fiber, and 7 grams of protein.

Beat the cream cheese and mayonnaise together until creamy, scraping the sides of the bowl often.

Add the Gouda, scallions, Parmesan, and pepper, and beat until well blended.

Chill, and serve with raw vegetables.

Avocado Cheese Dip

This dip has been known to make my mom a very popular person at parties. Dip with pork rinds, vegetables, or purchased protein chips. It can also be served over steak, and it makes perhaps the most elegant omelets on the face of the earth.

2 packages (8 ounces each) cream cheese, softened

1½ cups shredded white Cheddar or Monterey jack cheese

1 ripe black avocado, peeled and seeded

1 small onion

1 clove garlic, crushed

1 can (3 to 4 ounces) green chilies, drained, or jalapeños, if you like it hot

—

Yield: about 5 cups (plenty for a good-size party), with the batch containing 45 grams of carbohydrates and 9 grams of fiber, for a total of 36 grams of usable carbs and a whopping 83 grams of protein.

Combine all the ingredients in a food processor, and process until very smooth.

Scrape into a pretty serving bowl, and place the avocado seed in the middle.

WARNING

For some reason, placing the seed in the middle keeps the dip from turning brown quite so quickly while it sits out. But if you're making this a few hours ahead of time, cover it with plastic wrap, making sure the wrap is actually touching the surface of the dip. Don't make this more than a few hours before you plan to serve it.

Salty Ginger Pumpkin Seeds

Pumpkin seeds are terrific for you—they're a great source of both magnesium and zinc. And they taste great, too.

2 cups raw, shelled pumpkin seeds

2 tablespoons soy sauce

½ teaspoon powdered ginger

2 teaspoons Splenda

—

Yield: 4 servings, each with 13 grams of carbohydrates and 3 grams of fiber, for a total of 10 grams of usable carbs and 17 grams of protein. (These are also a terrific source of minerals.)

Preheat the oven to 350°F.

In a mixing bowl, combine the pumpkin seeds, soy sauce, ginger, and Splenda, mixing well.

Spread the pumpkin seeds in a shallow roasting pan, and roast for about 45 minutes, or until the seeds are dry, stirring two or three times during roasting.

Curried Pumpkin Seeds

You can actually buy curry-flavored pumpkin seeds, but these are bet-ter tasting and better for you.

4 tablespoons butter

2½ tablespoons curry powder

2 cloves garlic, crushed

2 cups raw, shelled pumpkin seeds

Salt

—

Yield: 4 servings, each with 15 grams of carbohydrates and 4 grams of fiber, for a total of 11 grams of usable carbs and 18 grams of protein.

Preheat the oven to 300°F.

Melt the butter in a small skillet over medium heat. Add the curry and garlic, and stir for 2 to 3 minutes.

In a mixing bowl, add the seasoned butter to the pumpkin seeds, and stir until well coated.

Spread the pumpkin seeds in a shallow roasting pan and roast for 30 minutes. Sprinkle lightly with salt.

WARNING

In addition to all the minerals found in the pumpkin seeds, you get the turmeric in the curry powder, which is believed to help prevent cancer.

Antipasto

This easy dish makes a nice light summer supper. Use some or all of the ingredients listed here, adjusting quantities as necessary.

Wedges of cantaloupe

Salami

Boiled ham

Pepperoncini (mildly hot salad peppers, available in jars near the pickles and olives)

Halved or quartered hard-boiled eggs

Marinated mushrooms

Black and green olives (get the good ones)

Strips of canned pimento

Solid-pack white tuna, drizzled with olive oil

Sardines

Marinated artichoke hearts (available in cans)

—

Yield: varies with your taste and needs, but here are the basic nutritional breakdowns for the items on your antipasto platter:

Simply arrange some or all of these things decoratively on a platter, put out a stack of small plates and some forks, and dinner is served.

CANTALOUPE, 1/8 of a small melon: 4.5 grams of carbohydrates and 0.5 grams of fiber, for a total of 4 grams of usable carbs and 0.5 grams of protein

SALAMI, 1 average slice: 0.5 grams of carbohydrates, a trace of fiber, and 3 grams of protein

BOILED HAM, 1 average slice: a trace of carbohydrates, no fiber, and 3.5 grams of protein

PEPPERONCINI, 1 average piece: 0.5 grams of carbohydrates, a trace of fiber, and no protein

HARD-BOILED EGGS, 1/2: 0.3 grams of carbohydrates, no fiber, and 3 grams of protein

MARINATED MUSHROOMS, 1 average piece: 1 gram of carbohydrates, a trace of fiber, and no protein

BLACK OLIVES, 1 large: 0.5 grams of carbohydrates, a trace of fiber, and no protein

GREEN OLIVES, 1 large: a trace of carbohydrates, a trace of fiber, and no protein

PIMENTO, 1 slice: a trace of carbohydrates, a trace of fiber, and no protein

TUNA, 3 ounces: no carbohydrates, no fiber, and 22 grams of protein

SARDINES, 2 average: no carbohydrates, no fiber, and 5 grams of protein (not to mention 91 milligrams of calcium)

ARTICHOKE HEARTS, 2 quarters: 2 grams of carbohydrates, 1 gram of fiber, and no protein

Maggie's Mushrooms

Lowcarbezine! reader Maggie Cosey sends this recipe.

1½ pounds large mushrooms

20 stuffed green olives

2 packages (8 ounces each) cream cheese, softened

⅛ to ¼ cup Worcestershire sauce

—

Yield: About 45 mushrooms, each with
1 gram of carbohydrates, a trace of fiber,
and 1 gram of protein.

Preheat the oven to 350°F.

Wash the mushrooms and remove their stems.

Chop the olives by hand or in a food processor.

In a mixing bowl, combine the olives, cream cheese, and Worcestershire sauce. (Be careful with the Worcestershire; there's a fine line between not enough and too much, it's better to err on the side of not enough.)

Spoon the mixture into the mushroom caps, and place them in a broiler pan.

Bake for 15 to 20 minutes, or until the cream cheese is slightly browned.

Simple Low-Carb Stuffed Mushrooms

1 pound medium mushrooms

1 pound bulk breakfast sausage, hot or sage

1 package (8 ounces) cream cheese

—

Yield: About 30 mushrooms, each with 1 gram of carbohydrates, a trace of fiber, and 3 grams of protein.

WASTE NOT, WANT NOT

If you freeze those stems and mushroom insides, you can use them for sautéed mushrooms the next time you have steak.

Preheat the oven to 350°F.

Clean the mushrooms. Remove their stems and use a paring knife to make the hole for stuffing larger.

Brown and drain the sausage, and stir in the cream cheese. Spoon the mixture into the mushroom caps.

Bake for 20 minutes.

Vicki's Crab-Stuffed Mushrooms

10 ounces medium portobello mushrooms

2 Wasa Fiber Rye crackers

1 can (6 ounces) crabmeat

1 egg

2 tablespoons lemon juice

1 tablespoon dried dill weed

1 teaspoon dehydrated onion flakes

½ cup grated Parmesan cheese

—

Yield: 6 appetizer-size servings, each with 4.5 grams of carbohydrates and 1 gram of fiber, for a total of 3.5 grams of usable carbs and 10 grams of protein.

Preheat the oven to 400°F.

Wipe the mushrooms clean with a damp cloth, and remove their stems. Set aside ½ cup of stems. Place the caps on an ungreased baking sheet.

Use a food processor with the S blade attached to grind the crackers into coarse crumbs. Add the ½ cup of mushroom stems, processing until coarsely chopped. Add the crabmeat, egg, lemon juice, dill, onion, and cheese. Mix thoroughly.

Spoon the mixture into the mushroom caps and bake for 12 to 15 minutes, or until the top of the stuffing is slightly browned. Serve hot.

Kay's Crab-Stuffed Mushrooms

These are for my cyberpal Kay, who repeatedly begged me to come up with a low-carb recipe for crab puffs. I tried and tried, but all my attempts were relatively pathetic. So I made crab-stuffed mushrooms instead, and they were a big hit.

1 pound fresh mushrooms

1 can (6½ ounces) flaked crab

2 ounces cream cheese

¼ cup mayonnaise

¼ cup grated Parmesan cheese

10 to 12 scallions, including the crisp part of the green shoot, finely sliced

Dash of Tabasco

¼ teaspoon pepper

—
Yield: 25 to 30 mushrooms, each with 1 gram of carbohydrates, a trace of fiber, and 3 grams of protein.

Preheat the oven to 325°F.

Wipe the mushrooms clean with a damp cloth, and remove their stems.

In a good-size bowl, combine the crab, cream cheese, mayonnaise, parmesan, scallions, Tabasco, and pepper well.

Spoon the mixture into the mushroom caps, and arrange them in a large, flat roasting pan.

Bake for 45 minutes to 1 hour, or until the mushrooms are done through. Serve hot (although folks will still scarf 'em down after they cool off).

WARNING

You may be tempted to make these with "fake crab" to save money. Don't. That stuff has a ton of carbohydrates added. Spend the extra couple of bucks and use real crab.

CHAPTER 3

Eggs, Dairy, and Breakfast Favorites

Before I get to the recipes, I'd like to urge you to stop thinking of eggs solely as a breakfast food. Eggs are wildly nutritious, infinitely versatile, they cook in a flash, and they're cheap, to boot. If you want a fast meal at any time of day, think eggs.

Omelets 101

There's this big mystique about omelets, maybe because they're a part of classic French cookery. People think that omelets are magically difficult and that only a true gourmet chef can get them right. But I say: Bah. Omelets are easy. Believe it or not, I've been known to turn out omelets for 20 on a propane camp stove. (This is when my friends started referring to my pop-up trailer as "Dana's House of Omelets.")

You can learn to do this quickly. Really—you can.

Before you begin, you'll need a good pan. What's a "good pan"? I prefer a 7-inch (medium-size) skillet with a heavy bottom, sloping sides, and a nonstick surface. However, what I currently have is a 7-inch skillet with a heavy bottom, sloping sides, and a formerly nonstick surface. I can still make omelets in it,—I just have to use a good shot of nonstick cooking spray. The heavy bottom and sloping sides, however, are essential.

Here's the really important thing to know about making omelets: The word "omelet" comes from a word meaning "to laminate," or to build up layers. And that's exactly what you do; you let a layer of beaten egg cook, then you lift up the edges and tip the pan so the raw egg runs under the cooked part. You do this all around the edges, of course, so you build it up evenly. The point is, you don't just let the beaten egg lie there in the skillet and wait for it to cook through. If you try to, the bottom will be hopelessly overdone before the top is set.

Dana's Easy Omelet Method

1. First, have your filling ready. If you're using vegetables, you'll want to sauté them first. If you're using cheese, have it grated or sliced and ready to go. If you're making an omelet to use up leftovers—a great idea, by the way—warm them through in the microwave and have them standing by.

2. Spray your omelet pan well with cooking spray if it doesn't have a good non-stick surface, and set it over medium-high heat.

3. While the skillet is heating, grab your eggs (two is the perfect number for this size pan, but one or three will work, too) and a bowl, crack the eggs, and beat them with a fork. Don't add water or milk or anything; just mix them up.

4. Test your pan to see if it's hot enough: A drop of water thrown in the pan should sizzle right away. Add a tablespoon of oil or butter, slosh it around to cover the bottom, then pour in the eggs, all at once. They should sizzle, too, and immediately start to set.

5. When the bottom layer of egg is set around the edges—and this should happen quite quickly—lift the edge using a spatula and tip the pan to let the raw egg flow underneath. Do this all around the edges, until there's not enough raw egg to run.

6. Turn your burner to the lowest heat if you have a gas stove. (If you have an electric stove, you'll have to have a "warm" burner standing by; electric elements don't cool off fast enough for this job.) Put your filling on one-half of the omelet, cover the pan with a lid, and let it sit over very low heat for a minute or two—no more. Peek and see if the raw, shiny egg is gone from the top surface (although you can serve it that way if you like; that's how the French prefer their omelets), and the cheese, if you've used it, is melted. If not, re-cover the pan and let it go another minute or two.

7. When your omelet is done, slip a spatula under the half without the filling, fold it over, and then lift the whole thing onto a plate. Or you can get fancy and tip the pan, letting the filling side of the omelet slide onto the plate and folding the top over as you go, but that takes some practice.

Cheese Omelet

This is pretty obvious, but you can't ignore a classic!

1 tablespoon butter

2 eggs, beaten

2 to 3 ounces sliced or shredded cheese (Cheddar, Monterey Jack, Colby, American, Swiss, Gruyère, Muenster, or whatever you prefer)

—

Yield: 1 serving, with 2 grams of carbohydrates, no fiber, and 32 grams of protein.

Make your omelet according to Dana's Easy Omelet Method (page 33), placing the cheese over half of your omelet when you get to step 6. Cover, turn the burner to low, and cook until the cheese is melted (2 to 3 minutes). Follow the directions to finish making the omelet.

Macro Cheese Omelet

My husband's favorite! With all that cheese, this is mighty filling.

1 tablespoon butter

2 eggs, beaten.

1 to 2 ounces Cheddar, sliced or shredded

1 to 2 ounces Monterey Jack, sliced or shredded

1 slice processed Swiss

—

Yield: 1 serving, with 3 grams of carbohydrates, no fiber, and 46 grams of protein.

Make your omelet according to Dana's Easy Omelet Method (page 33), placing the cheese over half of your omelet when you get to step 6. Cover, turn the burner to low, and cook until the cheese is melted (3 to 4 minutes). Follow the directions to finish making the omelet.

Taco Omelet

This is a great way to use up leftover taco filling.

1 tablespoon butter

2 eggs, beaten

¼ cup beef, turkey, or chicken taco filling, warmed.

2 tablespoons shredded Cheddar cheese

2 tablespoons salsa

1 tablespoon sour cream

—

Yield: 1 serving, with 3 grams of carbohydrates and 1 gram of fiber, for a total of 2 grams of usable carbs and 24 grams of protein. (Analysis does not include garnishes.)

Make your omelet according to Dana's Easy Omelet Method (page 33), placing the taco filling over half of your omelet when you get to step 6. Cover, turn the burner to low, and cook until the cheese is melted (3 to 4 minutes). Follow the directions to finish making the omelet. Sprinkle with the cheese, and top with salsa and sour cream.

> **NOTE**
>
> You can, if you like, jazz up this omelet with a little diced onion, olives, or whatever else you like on a taco.

Denver Omelet

1 tablespoon butter

2 eggs

1 ounce Cheddar cheese, shredded or sliced

¼ cup diced cooked ham

¼ green pepper, cut in small strips, sautéed

¼ small onion, sliced and sautéed

—

Yield: 1 serving, with 7 grams of carbohydrates and 1 gram of fiber, for a total of 6 grams of usable carbs (and you can cut that by using seriously low carb ham) and 25 grams of protein.

Make your omelet according to Dana's Easy Omelet Method (page 33), placing the cheese and the sautéed ham and vegetables over half of your omelet when you get to step 6. Cover, turn the burner to low, and cook until the cheese is melted (3 to 4 minutes). Follow the directions to finish making the omelet.

California Omelet

I've had breakfast down near the waterfront in San Diego. This is what it tastes like.

1 tablespoon olive oil

2 eggs, beaten

2 ounces Monterey Jack cheese, shredded

3 or 4 slices ripe avocado

¼ cup alfalfa sprouts

—

Yield: 1 serving with 4 grams of carbohydrates and 1 gram of fiber, for a total of 3 grams of usable carbs and 26 grams of protein (and as much potassium as a banana!).

Make your omelet according to Dana's Easy Omelet Method (page 33), placing the Monterey Jack over half of your omelet when you get to step 6. Cover, turn the burner to low, and cook until the cheese is melted (2 to 3 minutes). Arrange the avocado and sprouts over the cheese, and follow the directions to finish making the omelet.

New York Sunday Brunch Omelet

My husband was absolutely blown away by this. It's unbelievably filling, by the way.

1 tablespoon butter

2 eggs, beaten

2 ounces cream cheese, thinly sliced

¼ cup flaked smoked salmon

2 scallions, sliced

—

Yield: 1 serving with 5 grams of carbohydrates and 1 gram of fiber, for a total of 4 grams of usable carbs and 22 grams of protein.

Make your omelet according to Dana's Easy Omelet Method (page 33), placing the cream cheese over half of your omelet when you get to step 6. (Don't try to spread the cream cheese—it won't work!) Top with the salmon, cover, turn the burner to low, and cook until hot all the way through (2 to 3 minutes). Scatter the scallions over salmon, and follow the directions to finish making the omelet.

FRITTATAS

The frittata is the Italian version of the omelet, and it involves no folding! If you're still intimidated by omelets, try a frittata.

Confetti Frittata

¼ pound bulk pork sausage

¼ cup diced green pepper

¼ cup diced sweet red pepper

¼ cup diced sweet red onion

¼ cup grated Parmesan cheese

1 teaspoon Mrs. Dash, original flavor

8 eggs, beaten

—

Yield: 4 servings each with 4 grams of carbohydrates and 1 gram of fiber, for a total of 3 grams of usable carbohydrates and 17 grams of protein.

In a large, oven-proof skillet, start browning and crumbling the sausage over medium heat. As some fat starts to cook out of it, add the green peppers, red peppers, and onion to the skillet. Cook the sausage and veggies until there's no pink left in the sausage. Spread the sausage and veggie mixture into an even layer in the bottom of the skillet.

Beat the Parmesan cheese and Mrs. Dash into the eggs, and pour the mixture over the sausage and veggies in the skillet.

Turn the burner to low, and cover the skillet. (If your skillet doesn't have a cover, use foil.) Let the frittata cook until the eggs are mostly set. This will take 25 to 30 minutes, but the size of your skillet will affect the speed of cooking, so check periodically.

When all but the very top of the frittata is set, slide it under the broiler for about 5 minutes, or until the top is golden. Cut into wedges, and serve.

Artichoke Mushroom Frittata

Similar to the Artichoke Frittata on the opposite page, but adding mushrooms and leaving out the Parmesan cheese gives a whole new flavor.

3 tablespoons butter

1 cup canned, quartered artichoke hearts, drained

4 ounces fresh mushrooms, sliced

½ small onion, sliced

8 eggs, beaten

6 ounces shredded Gruyère cheese

—

Yield: 4 servings each with 7 grams of carbohydrates and 3 grams of fiber, for a total of 4 grams of usable carbs and 26 grams of protein.

In a heavy skillet, melt the butter and sauté the artichoke hearts, mushrooms, and onion over medium-low heat until the mushrooms are limp.

Spread the vegetables evenly over the bottom of the skillet, and pour the eggs over them.

Turn the burner to low, and cover the skillet. (If your skillet doesn't have a cover, use foil.) Let the frittata cook until mostly set (7 to 10 minutes).

Top with the Gruyère and slide the skillet under the broiler, about 4 inches from the heat. Broil for 2 to 3 minutes, or until the eggs are set on top and the cheese is lightly golden. Cut into wedges and serve.

SCRAMBLES

When both omelets and frittatas are too much trouble, just make a scramble. The ways of varying scrambled eggs are endless, so you could have them several times a week and never get bored. These have been analyzed assuming a three-egg serving, but if you want a lighter meal, leave out one egg and sub-tract 0.5 gram of carbohydrates and 6 grams of protein from my analysis.

Country Scramble

This fast-and-filling family-pleaser is a great way to use up leftover ham.

1 tablespoon butter

¼ cup diced cooked ham

¼ cup diced green pepper

2 tablespoons diced onion

3 eggs, beaten

Salt and pepper

—

Yield: 2 servings, each with 7 grams of carbohydrates and 1 gram of fiber, for a total of 6 grams of usable carbs and 23 grams of protein.

Melt the butter in a skillet over medium heat. Add the ham, green pepper, and onion, and sauté for a few minutes, until the onion is softened.

Pour in the eggs, and scramble until the eggs are set. Add salt and pepper to taste, and serve.

NOTE

Don't look at the number of servings and assume you can't feed a hungry family with a scramble—these recipes are a snap to double, as long as you have a skillet large enough to scramble in.

Italian Scramble

This is a good quick supper. Serve it with a green salad and some garlic bread for the kids.

2 tablespoons olive oil

¼ cup diced green pepper

¼ cup chopped onion

1 clove garlic, crushed

3 eggs

1 tablespoon grated Parmesan cheese

—

Yield: 1 serving, with 8 grams of carbohydrates and 1 gram of fiber, for a total of 7 grams of usable carbs and 17 grams of protein.

Heat the olive oil in a heavy skillet over medium heat, and sauté the pepper, onion, and garlic for 5 to 7 minutes, or until the onion is translucent.

Beat the eggs with the Parmesan, and pour into the skillet. Scramble until the eggs are set, and serve.

Mushroom Scramble

1 to 2 teaspoons butter

1 tablespoon minced onion

¼ cup sliced mushrooms

3 eggs, beaten

—

Yield: 1 serving, with 3 grams of carbohydrates, a trace of fiber, and 17 grams of protein.

Melt the butter in a heavy skillet over medium heat, and sauté the onion and mushrooms for 4 to 5 minutes, or until the mushrooms are tender.

Add the eggs, scramble until set, and serve.

FRIED EGGS

Tired of all that scrambling? These next few recipes are, in one form or another, good old fried eggs.

Fried Eggs Not Over Really Easy

If you're like me, you like your eggs over-easy, so that the whites are entirely set, but the yolks are still soft – but you find it maddeningly difficult to flip a fried egg without breaking the yolk. Here's the solution!

3 eggs
½ tablespoon butter or oil
1 teaspoon water

—
Yield: 1 serving, with about 1.5 grams of carbohydrates, no fiber, and 16 grams of protein.

NOTE

For the easiest eggs, use a skillet that fits the number of eggs you're frying. A 7-inch skillet is just right for a single serving, but if you're doing two servings, use a big skillet.

Spray your skillet with nonstick cooking spray, and place it over medium-high heat. When the skillet is hot, add the butter and coat the bottom of the pan with it. Crack your eggs into the skillet—careful not to break the yolks!—and immediately cover them.

Wait about 2 minutes, and check your eggs. They should be well set on the bottom, but still a bit slimy on top. Add a teaspoon of water for each serving (you can approximate this; the quantity isn't vital), turn the burner to low, and cover the pan again.

Check after a minute; the steam will have cooked the tops of the eggs. If there's still a bit of uncooked white, give it another 30 seconds to 1 minute. Lift out and serve.

Huevos Rancheros

1 tablespoon butter or oil

2 eggs

3 tablespoons salsa (hot or mild, as you prefer)

2 ounces Monterey Jack cheese, shredded

—

Yield: 1 serving, with 4 grams of carbohydrates and 1 gram of fiber, for a total of 3 grams of usable carbohydrates and 25 grams of protein.

Spray a heavy skillet with nonstick cooking spray, and set it over medium heat. Add the butter or oil, and crack the eggs into the skillet. Turn down the burner, and cover. Let the eggs fry for 4 to 5 minutes.

While the eggs are frying, warm the salsa in a saucepan or in the microwave.

When your fried eggs are set on the bottom but still a little underdone on top, scatter the cheese evenly over the fried eggs, add a teaspoon or two of water to the skil-let, and cover it again. In a minute or two, the tops of the eggs should be set (but the yolks still soft) and the cheese melted.

Transfer the eggs to a plate with a spatula, top with warmed salsa, and serve.

Rodeo Eggs

This was originally a sandwich recipe, but it works just as well without the bread.

4 slices bacon, chopped into 1-inch pieces

4 thin slices onion

4 eggs

4 thin slices Cheddar cheese

—

Yield: serves 2 if they're good and hungry or 4 if they're only a bit peckish, or if they're kids. In 2 servings, each will have 4 grams of carbohydrates, a trace of fiber, and 27 grams of protein.

Begin frying the bacon in a heavy skillet over medium heat. When some fat has cooked out of it, push it aside and put the onion slices in, too. Fry the onion on each side, turning carefully to keep the slices together, until it starts to look translucent. Remove the onion from the skillet, and set aside.

Continue frying the bacon until it's crisp. Pour off most of the grease, and distribute the bacon bits evenly over the bottom of the skillet. Break in the eggs and fry for a minute or two, until the bottoms are set but the tops are still soft. (If you like your yolks hard, break them with a fork; if you like them soft, leave them unbroken.)

Place a slice of onion over each yolk, then cover the onion with a slice of cheese. Add a teaspoon of water to the skillet, cover, and cook for 2 to 3 minutes, or until the cheese is thoroughly melted.

Cut into four separate eggs with the edge of a spatula, and serve.

Turkey Club Puff

Disguise your Friday-after-Thanksgiving leftovers in this delicious puff.

5 eggs

¼ cup soy powder or unflavored protein powder

½ teaspoon salt

½ teaspoon baking powder

1 cup cottage cheese

½ pound Swiss cheese, cubed

¼ cup melted butter

¾ cup cubed turkey

6 slices bacon, cooked until crisp

—

Yield: 5 servings, each with 5 grams of carbohydrates, a trace of fiber, and 33 grams of protein.

Preheat the oven to 350°F. Spray a 6-cup casserole with nonstick cooking spray, or butter generously.

Break the eggs into a bowl, and beat them with a whisk. Whisk in the soy powder, salt, and baking powder, mixing very well.

Beat in the cottage cheese, Swiss cheese, melted butter, cubed turkey and crumbled bacon. Pour the whole thing into the greased casserole. Bake for 35 to 40 minutes, or until set.

Sausage, Egg, and Cheese Bake

1 pound pork sausage (hot or mild, as you prefer)

½ cup diced green pepper

½ cup diced onion

8 eggs

¼ teaspoon pepper

1 cup shredded Cheddar cheese

1 cup shredded Swiss cheese

—

Yield: 6 servings, each with 4 grams of carbohydrates, a trace of fiber, and 26 grams of protein.

Preheat the oven to 350°F.

In a large, heavy, oven-proof skillet, start browning and crumbling the sausage over medium heat.

When some grease has cooked out of the sausage, add the green pepper and the onion, and continue cooking, stirring frequently, until the sausage is no longer pink.

In a large bowl, beat the eggs and pepper together, and stir in the Cheddar and Swiss cheeses.

Spread the sausage and vegetables evenly on the bottom of the skillet, and pour the egg and cheese mixture over it. Bake for 25 to 30 minutes, or until mostly firm but still just a little soft in the center.

Yogurt

When I tell people I make my own yogurt, they react as if I'd said I could transmute base metals into gold. But as you'll see, it's easy to make and considerably cheaper than buying the commercial stuff. "Officially," plain yogurt has 12 grams of carbohydrates per cup, but Dr. Goldberg and Dr. O'Mara point out in The GO-Diet that most of the lactose (milk sugar) is converted to lactic acid, leaving only about 4 grams per cup. So if you like yogurt, enjoy!

1 tablespoon plain yogurt

1½ to 2 cups instant dry milk, or a 1-quart envelope

> **NOTE**
>
> For your first batch, you'll use store-bought plain yogurt as a starter, but after that you can use a spoonful from the previous batch. Every so often it's good to start over with fresh, store-bought yogurt, though.

Fill a clean, 1-quart, snap-top container half full with water.

Put in the plain yogurt in the water, and stir. Add the powdered milk, and whisk until the lumps are gone.

Fill the container to the top with water, whisk it one last time, and put the lid on.

Put your yogurt-to-be in a warm place. I use a bowl lined with an old electric heating pad set on low, but any warm spot will do, such as inside an old-fashioned gas oven with a pilot light, on the stove top directly over the pilot light, or even near a heat register in winter.

Let your yogurt sit for 12 hours or so. It should be thick and creamy by then, but if it's still a little thin, give it a few more hours. When it's ready, stick it in the refrigerator and use it just like store-bought plain yogurt. Or flavor it with vanilla or lemon extract and some Splenda or stevia/FOS blend. You can also stir in a spoonful of sugar-free preserves, or mash a few berries with a fork and stir them in.

CHAPTER 4

Breads, Muffins, Cereals, and Other Grainy Things

Baked goods and other grain products, such as bread, cereal, pancakes, waffles, and so on, are among the foods that new low-carb dieters miss most. They are also among the foods that sell best for the low-carb specialty merchants. Many of these products are quite good, but they're often very pricey. With these recipes, you can make your own far more cheaply than you could buy them, and they'll often taste even better than the premade varieties available. When you know you can have a slice of toast or a grilled cheese sandwich now and then, your worries about your ability to stay low carb for the long haul will fade.

White Bread

This bread has a firm, fine texture and a great flavor.

1 cup water

¼ cup oat bran

2 tablespoons psyllium husks

¾ cup vital wheat gluten

½ cup vanilla-flavored whey protein powder

⅓ cup rice protein powder

1 teaspoon salt

1 tablespoon oil

1 tablespoon Splenda

2 teaspoons yeast

—
Yield: About 10 slices, each with 5 grams
of carbohydrates and 1 gram of fiber, for a total
of 4 grams of usable carbs and 24 grams of protein.

Put the ingredients in your bread machine in the order given, and run the machine. Remove the loaf from the machine and bread case promptly to cool.

"Whole Wheat" Bread

Slice this extra-thin so you can "afford" two slices, and it makes a great grilled cheese sandwich.

½ cup warmwater

½ cup heavy cream

1 tablespoon soft butter

1 egg

1 teaspoon salt

¾ cup vital wheat gluten

2 tablespoons raw wheat germ

2 tablespoons wheat bran

¼ cup psyllium husks

½ cup oat flour

½ cup vanilla-flavored whey protein powder

2 teaspoons yeast

—

Yield: About 10 slices, each with 13 grams of carbohydrates and 7.5 grams of fiber, for a total of 5.5 grams of usable carbs and 19 grams of protein (more than two eggs!).

Put the ingredients in your bread machine in the order given, and run the machine. Remove the loaf from the machine and bread case promptly to cool.

Cinnamon Raisin Bread

Sweet and cinnamony! Have a slice of this toasted and slathered with butter for breakfast, and you'll never know you're on a low-carb diet!

¾ cup plus 2 tablespoons warm water

¼ cup oat bran

½ cup ground almonds

⅓ cup vanilla-flavored whey protein powder

1½ teaspoons cinnamon

¾ cup plus 3 tablespoons vital wheat gluten

¼ cup Splenda

1 tablespoon oil

1 teaspoon salt

2 teaspoons yeast

2 tablespoons raisins, each snipped in half

—
Yield: 12 slices, each with 6 grams of carbohydrates and 0.6 grams of fiber, for a total of 5.4 grams of usable carbs and 19 grams of protein.

Put the ingredients in your bread machine in the order given, and run the machine. Remove the loaf from the machine and bread case promptly to cool.

NOTE

The reason you cut the raisins in half is to let them distribute more evenly throughout the bread; even so, there aren't a lot of them, I'll admit. That's because the raisins are the highest-carb part of this bread. If you want, you can leave them whole so each one will be more noticeable.

Heart-y Bread

So named because both rice bran and flax are known to lower cholesterol. Want more good news? This bread tastes as good as it is good for you.

1 cup plus 2 tablespoons water

⅓ cup rice bran

⅓ cup flaxseed meal

1 cup vital wheat gluten

⅓ cup vanilla-flavored whey protein powder

2 teaspoons blackstrap molasses

1 teaspoon salt

1 tablespoon oil

2 teaspoons yeast

—
Yield: 11 slices, each with 6.7 grams of carbohydrates and 2.6 grams of fiber, for a total of 4.1 grams of usable carbs and 19 grams of protein.

Put the ingredients in your bread machine in the order given, and run the machine. Remove the loaf from the machine and bread case promptly to cool.

French Toast

Make this for breakfast some lazy weekend morning, and the family will think you're cheating on your diet!

4 eggs

½ cup heavy cream

½ cup water

1 teaspoon vanilla extract (optional)

6 slices low-carb bread of your choice (white, "whole wheat," cinnamon raisin, and oatmeal molasses are all good choices)

Butter

—

Yield: 6 servings. The carb count will vary with the type of bread you use, but the egg and cream add only 2 grams of carbs, no fiber, and 4 grams of protein per slice.

Beat together the eggs, heavy cream, water, and vanilla extract (if using), and place the mixture in a shallow dish, such as a pie plate.

Soak the slices of bread in the mixture until they're well saturated; you'll have to do them one or two at a time. Let each slice soak for at least 5 minutes, turning once.

Fry each soaked piece of bread in plenty of butter over medium heat in a heavy skillet or griddle. Brown well on each side.

Serve with sugar-free syrup, cinnamon and Splenda, or sugar-free preserves, as you choose.

Evelyn's Granola

From reader Evelyn Nordahl, a much lower-carbohydrate granola recipe.

1 cup Textured Vegetable Protein granules

1 teaspoon cinnamon

2 tablespoons Splenda

½ cup unsweetened coconut flakes

½ cup chopped pecans

½ cup chopped, sliced, or slivered almonds

—

Yield: About 10 servings of ¼ cup, each with 9 grams of carbohydrates and 6 grams of fiber, for a total of 3 grams of usable carbs and 17 grams of protein.

Combine the Textured Vegetable Protein granules, cinnamon, and Splenda in a plastic or glass container large enough to hold all the ingredients.

Spread the coconut, pecans, and almonds on a cookie sheet and toast under the broiler just until the coconut starts to brown. Remove from the oven and cool.

Add the toasted nuts to the granule mixture, attach the lid, and shake to mix.

NOTE

Evelyn eats this granola topped with about 2 tablespoons of water and 2 tablespoons of heavy cream, and she says it's "satisfying, crunchy and delicious."

English Muffins

Yes, you can make your own low-carb English Muffins. The yogurt is what gives them that characteristic, mildly sour taste.

½ cup warm water

½ cup yogurt

1 teaspoon salt

⅔ cup vital wheat gluten

¼ cup psyllium husks

2 tablespoons raw wheat germ

¼ cup wheat bran

½ cup oat flour

½ cup vanilla-flavored whey protein powder

1½ teaspoons yeast

—
Yield: About 6 muffins, or 12 servings,
each with 13 grams of carbohydrates and 6.5 grams of fiber, for a total of 6.5 grams of usable carbs and 14 grams of protein.

Put the ingredients in your bread machine in the order given, and run until the end of the "rise" cycle. Remove the dough from the machine.

Using just enough oat flour on your work surface to keep the dough from sticking, pat the dough out so it's ½ inch thick.

Using a tin can with both ends removed as a cutter (a tuna can works well), cut rounds from the dough. Cover them with a clean cloth, set them aside in a warm place, and let them rise for about 1 hour, or until they've doubled in bulk.

Heat a heavy skillet or griddle over medium-low heat. Scatter the surface lightly with wheat germ to prevent sticking, and place as many muffins in the skillet as will fit easily. Let the muffins bake for about 6 minutes per side, or until they're browned. Eat these just like you would regular English muffins—split them, toast them, and butter them.

Granola

This isn't super-low in carbs, and it's really more for eating during maintenance than during weight loss. But it's far lower in carbs than standard granola, high in protein, very filling, and best of all, it tastes like real cereal!

2½ cups rolled oats

¾ cup sunflower seeds

¾ cup sesame seeds

⅔ cup wheat germ

¾ cup flaked, unsweetened coconut

½ cup chopped walnuts

½ cup slivered almonds

½ cup wheat bran

¼ cup flaxseeds

1 teaspoon cinnamon

½ cup Splenda

¾ cup vanilla-flavored whey protein powder

¼ teaspoon blackstrap molasses

½ cup canola oil

—

Yield: Makes about 16 servings of ½ cup, each with 21.8 grams of carbohydrates and 6 grams of fiber, for a total of 15.8 grams of usable carbs and 11.6 grams of protein.

Preheat the oven to 250°F.

In a large, shallow roasting pan, combine the rolled oats, sunflower seeds, sesame seeds, wheat germ, coconut, walnuts, almonds, bran, flaxseeds, cinnamon, Splenda, and protein powder, mixing them very well.

Stir the molasses into the canola oil; it won't really blend with it, but it will help the molasses get distributed evenly. Pour the mixture over the dry ingredients, and stir until it's uniformly distributed.

Place in the oven and toast for an hour, stirring once or twice. Store in a tightly covered container. Serve topped with cream or half-and-half.

Almond Pancake and Waffle Mix

This makes nice, tender pancakes and waffles that have a nutty taste and a texture similar to cornmeal pancakes and waffles.

2 cups almond meal

½ cup oat bran

½ cup vanilla-flavored whey protein powder

½ cup rice protein powder

2 tablespoons wheat bran

2 tablespoons raw wheat germ

2 tablespoons vital wheat gluten

2½ tablespoons baking powder

1½ teaspoons salt

—

Yield: Makes about 4 servings of 1 cup, each with 33 grams of carbohydrates and 3 grams of fiber, for a total of 30 grams of usable carbs and 36 grams of protein.

Assemble all the ingredients in a food processor with the S blade in place. Run the processor for a minute or so, stopping once or twice to shake it so everything will be well combined.

Store the mix in an airtight container in the refrigerator.

Pancakes from Almond Mix

I like to eat these topped with sugar-free grape jelly, but you could also serve them with sugar-free syrup, sugar-free jam, thawed sugar-free frozen fruit, or Splenda and cinnamon.

2 cups Almond Pancake and Waffle Mix
(see above)

2 eggs

1 cup water

1 tablespoon canola, peanut, or sunflower oil

—

Yield: About 16 pancakes, each with 4 grams of carbohydrates, a trace of fiber, and 6 grams of protein.

Spray a skillet or griddle with nonstick cooking spray, and set it over medium heat.

Mix all the ingredients with a whisk, and drop the batter by the tablespoonful onto the griddle or skillet. Cook as you would regular pancakes, turning to brown lightly on each side. Stir the batter between batches to prevent it from settling.

NOTE

For a little added flavor, melt a little butter on the griddle or skillet before you cook the batter.

Waffles from Almond Mix

These remind me a lot of cornmeal waffles, and they're really good with bacon on the side.

1 cup Almond Pancake and Waffle Mix
(see page 53)

1 teaspoon Splenda

½ cup half-and-half

1 egg

¼ cup oil

—
**Yield: In my waffle iron, this makes
6 servings,** each with 5 grams of carbohydrates,
a trace of fiber, and 6 grams of protein.

Preheat a waffle iron.

In a mixing bowl, stir together the mix and Splenda.

In a separate bowl, stir together the half-and-half, egg, and oil, and pour the mixture into the dry ingredients. Stir only until everything is wet, and there are no big lumps of dry mix.

Bake in the waffle iron according to the machine's directions. Serve with butter and sugar-free syrup, cinnamon and Splenda, sugar-free jam or jelly, or another low-carb topping of your choice.

Sunflower Parmesan Crackers

These have a great, crunchy texture and a wonderful flavor.

1 cup raw, shelled sunflower seeds

½ cup grated Parmesan cheese

¼ cup water

—

Yield: How many carbs per cracker? It will vary with the size and thickness of your crackers. I get about 6 dozen, each with just a trace of carbohydrates, a trace of fiber, and 1 gram of protein. But you can eat the whole batch for just 13 grams of usable carbohydrates, so who's counting?

ABOUT MAKING LOW-CARB CRACKERS

To make all these cracker recipes, you will need a roll of nonstick baking parchment, available at housewares stores everywhere, or Teflon pan liners, available at really good cookware stores. My roll of baking parchment cost me all of $3. Do not try to simply make these crackers on a cookie sheet, no matter how well greased: As you stand at your sink, endlessly, laboriously chipping your crackers off the cookie sheet, you will be very sorry.

Preheat the oven to 325°F.

Put the sunflower seeds and Parmesan in a food processor with the S blade in place, and process until the sunflower seeds are a fine meal with almost a flour consistency. Add the water, and pulse the processor until the dough is well blended, soft, and sticky.

Cover your cookie sheet with a piece of baking parchment. Turn the dough out onto the parchment, tear off another sheet of parchment, and put it on top of the dough.

Through the top sheet of parchment, use your hands to press the dough into as thin and even a sheet as you can. Take the time to get the dough quite thin—the thinner, the better, so long as there are no holes in the dough. Peel off the top layer of parchment, and use a thin, sharp, straight-bladed knife or a pizza cutter to score the dough into squares or diamonds.

Bake for about 30 minutes, or until evenly browned. Peel off the parchment, break along the scored lines, and let the crackers cool. Store them in a container with a tight lid.

PIZZA

A big thank you to Jennifer Eloff for this recipe from Splendid Low-Carbing!
*To make these pizza crusts, you first have to make her Almond Whey Bake
Mix #1.*

Almond Whey Bake Mix #1

1⅓ cups ground almonds

¾ cup natural whey protein powder

½ cup unbleached spelt flour or ½ cup
unbleached all-purpose flour

1 tablespoon vital wheat gluten

In a medium bowl, combine all the ingredients
and stir well. Store in an airtight
container at room temperature.

Whey Pizza Crusts

Now, use the bake mix to make your Pizza Crusts.

¾ cup water, less 1 tablespoon

2 tablespoons olive oil

1½ cups Almond Whey Bake Mix #1
(see page 56)

⅔ cup vital wheat gluten

½ cup wheat bran

⅓ cup natural whey protein powder

2 tablespoons Splenda

1 tablespoon spelt flour or all-purpose flour

1 tablespoon sugar

1 tablespoon skim milk powder

1 tablespoon bread machine yeast

1 teaspoon salt

—
**Yield: 2 pizzas with 12 slices each,
or 24 servings.** The carb count of your toppings
will vary, depending on what you use, but the crust
will add just 2.6 grams of carbohydrates, no fiber,
and 6 grams of protein.

NOTE

A convection oven bakes pizza evenly
and more quickly, so be sure to adjust
your baking time accordingly.

Preheat the oven to 375°F, and warm the water in
the microwave for 30 seconds.

Place the water, olive oil, Bake Mix #1, wheat
gluten, wheat bran, protein powder, Splenda, flour,
sugar, skim milk powder, yeast, and salt in the bread
machine.

Program the bread machine for pizza dough, or
knead and first rise.

When the dough is ready, remove it from the
machine and divide it in half. On a lightly floured
surface, roll out each ball of dough as far as possible.
Cover with a towel, and allow to sit for 10 to 20
minutes. Grease two 12-inch pizza pans.

Roll the dough again. Place it on the pizza pans,
and roll it out to fit each pan, using a small rolling
pin or another small cylindrical object.

Cover the crusts with pizza sauce, toppings, and
grated cheese. Bake on lowest oven rack for 20 to
25 minutes, or until the crusts are browned.

TORTILLAS

Yet another great recipe from Splendid Low-Carbing *by Jennifer Eloff.*
Again, you start this recipe by making a bake mix:

Almond Whey Bake Mix #2

1⅓ cup ground almonds

¾ cup spelt flour

½ cup natural whey protein powder

¼ cup vital wheat gluten

In a medium bowl, combine all ingredients. Mix with a wooden spoon until well combined. Store in an airtight container.

Whey Tortillas

Jen Eloff at sweety.com says, "These, in my humble opinion, taste better than the regular, almost tasteless white flour tortillas we used to buy."

¾ cup warm water (105° to 115°F; this will feel warm, but not hot, on your wrist)

1 tablespoon sugar

1 tablespoon yeast

2 tablespoons olive oil

1⅓ cups Almond Whey Bake Mix #2 (see page 58)

⅔ cup vital wheat gluten

½ cup wheat bran

⅓ cup spelt flour or all-purpose flour

2 tablespoons Splenda

1 tablespoon sugar

1 tablespoon skim milk powder

1 teaspoon salt

—

Yield: 20 tortillas, each with 4.4 grams of carbohydrates, no fiber. and 6.2 grams of protein.

Preheat the oven to 200°F.

Pour the warm water in a large electric mixer bowl. Dissolve the sugar in the water, and then sprinkle yeast over the water's surface.

Allow the mixture to sit for 3 to 5 minutes, then stir to dissolve completely.

Add the olive oil, Almond Whey Bake Mix #2, wheat gluten, wheat bran, flour, Splenda, sugar, skim milk powder, and salt. Using a dough hook attachment on an electric mixer, mix, scraping the sides of the bowl occasionally, until the dough is moist and elastic. (If you don't have an electric mixer, you can do this by hand, with a wooden spoon.)

On a lightly floured surface, knead the dough briefly, and then place it in a greased bowl. Cover loosely with foil and place it in the oven. Turn the oven off, and allow the dough to double in size (this will take about 1 hour).

When the dough has risen, remove, punch down, and break into 20 small balls. Cover the dough balls with a clean dishtowel to keep them from drying out.

Roll each dough ball into a paper-thin circle on a lightly floured surface.

In a dry, nonstick skillet, cook each dough round briefly on both sides, until brown spots appear. Place your tortillas in a plastic bag to keep them supple, or refrigerate or freeze for longer storage.

CHAPTER 5

Hot Vegetable Dishes

When folks first go low–carb, they suddenly don't know what to serve for side dishes. The answer is vegetables. If you're used to thinking of vegetables as something that sits between the meat and the potato, usually being ignored, read this chapter and think again! You'll notice a certain reliance on frozen vegetables in this chapter. I confess, I use them often, especially green beans and broccoli. The convenience is worth it to me, and I think the quality is good. Feel free to use fresh, if you like, remembering that they'll take a few more minutes to cook.

Fauxtatoes Deluxe

This extra-rich fauxtatoes recipe comes from Adele Hite of Eathropology.com, and it is the basis for the "grits" part of her Low-Carb Shrimp and "Grits" recipe (page 204). Adele suggests, "Give your Fauxtatoes a little zing by adding a few cloves of sliced garlic to the cooking water or some roasted garlic to the food processor when blending the cauliflower with the other ingredients. Each clove of garlic added will add just 1 gram of carbohydrates to the carb count for the batch."

1 large head cauliflower

⅓ cup cream

4 ounces cream cheese

1 tablespoon butter

Salt and pepper

—

Yield: 6 generous servings, each with 6 grams of carbohydrates and 2 grams of fiber, for a total of 4 grams of usable carbs and 4 grams of protein.

Simmer the cauliflower in water with the cream added to it. (This keeps the cauliflower sweet and prevents it from turning an unappetizing gray color.) When the cauliflower is very soft, drain thoroughly.

Put the still-warm cauliflower in a food processor with the cream cheese, butter, and salt and pepper to taste, and process until smooth. (You may have to do this in more than one batch.)

NOTE

Give your fauxtatoes a little zing by adding a few cloves of sliced garlic to the cooking water or some roasted garlic to the food processor when blending the cauliflower with the other ingredients. Each clove of garlic added will add just 1 gram of carbohydrates to the carb count for the batch.

Cauliflower Rice

Many thanks to Fran McCullough! I got this idea from her book *Living Low Carb,* and it's served me very well.

½ head cauliflower

—

Yield: about 3 cups, or 3 servings, each with 5 grams of carbohydrates and 2 grams of fiber, for a total of 3 grams of usable carbs and 2 grams of protein.

Simply put the cauliflower through your food processor using the shredding blade. This gives the cauliflower a texture that's remarkably similar to rice. You can steam, microwave, or even sauté it in butter. Whatever you do, though, don't overcook it!

Cauliflower Rice Deluxe

This is higher-carb than plain Cauliflower Rice, but the wild rice adds a grain flavor that makes it quite convincing. Plus, wild rice has about 25 percent less carbohydrates than most other kinds of rice. I only use this for special occasions, but it's wonderful.

3 cups Cauliflower Rice (see page 61)

¼ cup wild rice

¾ cup water

—

Yield: 4 cups, or 8 servings, each with 6 grams of carbohydrates and 1 gram of fiber, for a total of 5 grams of usable carbs and 2 grams of protein.

Cook your cauliflower rice as desired (I steam mine when making this), taking care not to overcook it to mushiness, but just until it's tender.

Put the wild rice and water in a saucepan, cover it, and set it on a burner on lowest heat until all the water is gone (at least one-half hour, maybe a bit more).

Toss together the cooked cauliflower rice and wild rice, and season as desired.

Company Dinner "Rice"

This is my favorite way to season the cauliflower–wild rice blend above. It's a big hit at dinner parties!

1 small onion, chopped

1 stick butter, melted

4 cups Cauliflower Rice Deluxe (see above)

6 strips bacon, cooked until crisp, and crumbled

¼ teaspoon salt or Vege-Sal

¼ teaspoon pepper

½ cup grated Parmesan cheese

—

Yield: 8 servings, each with 8 grams of carbohydrates and 2 grams of fiber, for a total of 6 grams of usable carbs and 5 grams of protein.

Sauté the onion in the butter until it's golden and limp. Toss the Cauliflower Rice Deluxe with the sautéed onion and the bacon, salt, pepper, and cheese. Serve.

Ratatouille

You pronounce this oh-so-French dish "rat-a-TOO-ee."

¾ cup olive oil

3 cups chopped eggplant, cut into 1-inch cubes

3 cups sliced zucchini

1 medium onion, sliced

2 green peppers, cut into strips

3 cloves garlic

1 can (14½ ounces) sliced tomatoes

1 can (4 ounces) sliced black olives, drained

1½ teaspoons dried oregano

½ teaspoon salt

¼ teaspoon pepper

—
Yield: 8 servings, each with 11 grams of carbohydrates and 3 grams of fiber, for a total of 8 grams of usable carbs and 2 grams of protein.

Heat the oil in a heavy skillet over medium heat. Add the eggplant, zucchini, onion, peppers, and garlic.

Sauté for 15 to 20 minutes, turning with a spatula from time to time so it all comes in contact with the olive oil. Once the vegetables are all starting to look about half-cooked, add the tomatoes (including the liquid), olives, oregano, salt, and pepper.

Stir it all together, cover, turn the burner to low, and let the whole thing simmer for 40 minutes or so.

NOTE

You want to use your largest skillet for this dish—possibly even your wok, if you have one. This amount of veggies will cause even a 10-inch skillet to nearly overflow. And don't be afraid to toss in a little more olive oil if you need it while sautéing.

Buttered Snow Peas

If you've only had snow peas in Chinese food, try them this way. They're really wonderful.

4 tablespoons butter

12 ounces fresh snow peas

—

Yield: 3 servings, each with 9 grams of carbohydrates and 3 grams of fiber, for a total of 6 grams of usable carbs and 3 grams of protein.

Melt the butter in a heavy skillet over medium-high heat.

Add the snow peas, and sauté just until tender-crisp.

About Cooking Asparagus

Asparagus is divine if cooked correctly, and mushy and nasty if overcooked—and it's way too easy to overcook. If you're cooking it on the stove top, the best way, believe it or not, is standing up in an old stove top coffee perker with the guts removed. This lets the tougher ends boil while the tender tips steam. I put my asparagus in the coffee pot, add about 3 inches of water, and put on the lid. Set it over a medium-high burner, and bring the water to a boil. Once it's boil-ing, 5 minutes is plenty!

If you don't have a coffee perker (or an asparagus pot, for that matter, which lets you do the same thing), I'd recommend that you microwave your asparagus. Place the stems in a microwave-safe casserole or glass pie plate. If you're using a pie plate or a round casserole, arrange the asparagus with the tips toward the center. (I've microwaved asparagus in a rectangular casserole, and it's come out fine.) Add a tablespoon or two of water, and cover with plastic wrap or a lid, if your casserole has one. Microwave it on High for 5 to 6 minutes, then remove the plastic wrap or lid immediately, or the trapped steam will keep cooking your asparagus.

One more asparagus note: Believe it or not, the proper way to eat asparagus is with your fingers, dipping it in whatever sauce may be provided. This is according to Miss Manners, Amy Vanderbilt, and all other etiquette authorities. It's definitely more fun than using a fork—the kids may even take to asparagus this way—and it's amusing to see people look at you, thinking, "With her fingers?" knowing all along that you are correct and they are incorrect.

Asparagus with Lemon Butter

To me, this is the taste of springtime.

1 pound asparagus

¼ cup butter

1 tablespoon lemon juice

—

Yield: 4 servings, each with 5 grams of carbohydrates and 2 grams of fiber, for a total of 3 grams of usable carbs and 3 grams of protein.

Break the ends off the asparagus where they snap naturally. Steam or microwave the asparagus until just barely tender-crisp.

While the asparagus is cooking, melt the butter and stir in the lemon juice. Put the lemon butter in a pretty little pitcher, and let each diner pour a pool of it onto his or her plate for dipping.

Creamed Spinach

1 package (10 ounces) frozen, chopped spinach, thawed

¼ cup heavy cream

¼ cup grated Parmesan cheese

1 clove garlic, crushed

—

Yield: 3 servings, each with 5 grams of carbohydrates and 3 grams of fiber, for a total of 2 grams of usable carbs and 6 grams of protein.

Put all the ingredients in a heavy-bottomed saucepan over medium-low heat, and simmer for 7 to 8 minutes.

Greek Spinach

1 tablespoon butter

¼ small onion, minced

1 package (10 ounces) frozen, chopped spinach, thawed

¼ cup crumbled feta cheese

¼ cup cottage cheese

—

Yield: 3 servings, each with 6 grams of carbohydrates and 3 grams of fiber, for a total of 3 grams of usable carbs and 7 grams of protein.

Melt the butter in a heavy skillet over medium heat. Add the onion, and let it sizzle for just a minute. Add the spinach and sauté, stirring now and then, for 5 to 7 minutes.

Add in the cheeses and stir until they start to melt. Let the spinach cook for another minute or so, then serve.

Sag Paneer

With cottage cheese, this isn't totally authentic, but it's mighty tasty.

2 tablespoons butter

1 teaspoon curry powder

1 package (10 ounces) frozen, chopped spinach, thawed

1 teaspoon salt or Vege-Sal

⅓ cup small-curd cottage cheese

2 teaspoons sour cream

—

Yield: 3 servings, each with 5 grams of carbohydrates and 3 grams of fiber, for a total of 2 grams of usable carbs and 6 grams of protein.

Melt the butter in a heavy skillet over low heat, and stir in the curry powder. Let the curry powder cook in the butter for 3 to 4 minutes.

Stir in the spinach and the salt. Cover the skillet, and let the spinach cook for 4 to 5 minutes, or until heated through.

Stir in the cottage cheese and sour cream, and cook, stirring, until the cheese has completely melted.

About Cooking Broccoli

If you're using fresh broccoli, cut it up and peel the stems. If you've been discarding the stems, you'll be startled to discover that they're the best part of the broccoli once you've peeled off the tough skin.

Broccoli is another vegetable that's great when it's cooked just barely enough, but revolting when it's overcooked. I often think that the reason there are so many broccoli-haters in the world is because they've only been exposed to mushy, sulfurous, gray, overcooked broccoli. So above all, don't overcook your broccoli!

You can steam or microwave broccoli interchangeably. If you're steaming, start timing after the water comes to a boil. Fresh broccoli needs about 7 minutes and frozen broccoli (assuming you start with it still frozen) needs 10 or 11 minutes. If you're microwaving your broccoli (my favorite way to cook it), put it in a microwave-safe casserole, add a tablespoon or two of water, and cover with plastic wrap or a lid. Microwave on High for about 5 minutes for fresh broccoli or closer to 10 minutes for frozen, stirring halfway through to make sure it cooks evenly. However you cook your broccoli, uncover it as soon as it reaches the degree of doneness you prefer, or it will continue to cook and end up mushy.

Broccoli with Lemon Butter

I'm always bemused when I see frozen broccoli with lemon butter at the grocery store. I mean, how hard is it to add butter and lemon juice to your broccoli?

1 pound frozen broccoli or 1 large head fresh broccoli

4 tablespoons butter

1 tablespoon lemon juice

—

Yield: 4 servings, each with 6 grams of carbohydrates and 3 grams of fiber, for a total of 3 grams of usable carbs and 3 grams of protein.

Steam or microwave your broccoli. When it's cooked, drain off the water, and toss the broccoli with the butter and lemon juice until the butter is melted. That's it!

About Cooking Spaghetti Squash

If you've never cooked a spaghetti squash, you may be puzzled as to how to go about it, but it's really easy: Just stab it several times (to keep it from exploding), and put it in your microwave on High for 12 to 15 minutes. Then slice it open, and scoop out and discard the seeds. Now take a fork and start scraping at the "meat" of the squash. You will be surprised and charmed to discover that it separates into strands very much like spaghetti, only yellow-orange in color.

Spaghetti squash is not a terribly low-carb vegetable, but it's much lower-carb than spaghetti, so it's a useful substitute in many recipes—especially casseroles. If you only need half of your cooked spaghetti squash right away, the rest will live happily in a zipper-lock bag in your fridge for 3 to 4 days until you do something else with it.

Spaghetti Squash Alfredo

We love this! My husband is an Alfredo fiend, so by using spaghetti squash instead of pasta, he gets his fix without all those additional carbs.

2 cups cooked spaghetti squash

3 tablespoons butter

3 tablespoons heavy cream

1 clove garlic, crushed

¼ cup grated or shredded Parmesan cheese

—

Yield: 4 servings, each with 4 grams of carbohydrates, a trace of fiber, and 3 grams of protein.

Simply heat up your squash, and stir in everything else. Stir until the butter is melted, and serve!

NOTE

This makes a very nice side dish with some chicken sautéed in olive oil and garlic.

Spaghetti Squash Carbonara

This makes a very filling side dish.

8 slices bacon

4 eggs

¾ cup grated Parmesan cheese

3 cups cooked spaghetti squash

1 clove garlic, crushed

—
Yield: 6 servings, each with 6 grams of carbohydrates and 1 gram of fiber, for a total of 5 grams of usable carbs and 11 grams of protein.

NOTE

You can make this dish higher in protein by using a cup or two of diced, leftover ham in place of the bacon. Brown the ham in olive oil, remove from the pan, cook the squash mixture in the oil, and then toss in the ham just before serving.

Fry the bacon until it's crisp. Remove from pan, and pour off all but a couple tablespoons of grease.

Beat the eggs with the cheese, and toss with the spaghetti squash. Pour the squash mixture into the hot fat in the skillet, and add the garlic. Toss for 2 to 3 minutes.

Crumble in the bacon, toss, and serve.

Spicy Sesame "Noodles" with Vegetables

This isn't terribly low-carb, but it sure can pull you out of the hole when you've got vegetarians coming to dinner.

3 cups cooked spaghetti squash

¼ cup water

3 tablespoons soy sauce

5 tablespoons tahini

1½ tablespoons rice vinegar

½ teaspoon red pepper flakes

1 tablespoon sesame seeds

2 to 3 tablespoons peanut oil or other bland oil

1½ cups mushrooms, thickly sliced

⅔ cup diced green pepper

½ cup diced celery

½ cup chopped onion

¼ pound snow peas, cut into 1-inch lengths

2 tablespoons grated fresh ginger

2 cloves garlic, crushed

½ cup cooked shrimp or diced leftover chicken, pork, or ham per serving (optional)

—

Yield: 4 servings, each with 19 grams of carbohydrates and 4 grams of fiber, for a total of 15 grams of usable carbs and 7 grams of protein. (Analysis does not include optional meat.)

NOTE

This is a great dish to make for guests, because so much of it can be done ahead of time: You can prepare the noodles (step 2) and the garnish (step 3) before your company arrives, and then just stir-fry the veggies and garnish the plates when it's time to eat.

Place the spaghetti squash in a large mixing bowl.

In a separate bowl, combine the water, soy sauce, tahini, rice vinegar, and pepper flakes, mixing well. Pour over the spaghetti squash, and set aside.

Place your sesame seeds in a small, heavy skillet over high heat, and shake the skillet constantly until the seeds start to "pop." They won't pop like popcorn, but they will make little popping sounds and jump in the skillet. When that happens, immediately turn off the heat and shake the seeds out onto a small plate to cool. Set aside.

Just before you're ready to serve the dish, heat the oil in a large skillet or wok. Add the mushrooms, pepper, celery, onion, snow peas, ginger, and garlic, and stir-fry over high heat for 7 to 10 minutes or until tender-crisp.

When the vegetables are done, add them to the large mixing bowl with the spaghet-ti squash mixture, and toss until well combined.

Pile the veggies and "noodles" on serving plates. Top the meat-eaters' servings with the shrimp, chicken, pork, or ham (if using), and scatter sesame seeds over each serving.

CHAPTER 6

Poultry Mains

Around here we eat chicken no fewer than a couple of times a week, and many other families do the same. After all, chicken is inexpensive, and it's always tasty. It also lends itself to infinite variation, as this chapter will prove. Until fairly recently, you could buy a cut-up broiler-fryer—a package with two breasts with wings attached and two leg-and-thigh quarters. This is what my mother always bought because some of us liked white meat and some of us—me included—preferred dark. Sadly, the cut-up broiler-fryer no longer appears in my grocery stores. Instead we have packages of just breasts, wings, thighs, drumsticks, etc. I feel this is a shame, but most people must prefer it, or it wouldn't have taken over the market.

Tarragon Chicken

1 cut up broiler-fryer

2 tablespoons butter

1 teaspoon salt or Vege-Sal

Pepper

3 tablespoons dried tarragon

1 clove garlic, crushed

½ cup dry white wine

—

Yield: 4 servings, each with 2 grams of carbohydrates, a trace of fiber, and 44 grams of protein.

If your chicken is in quarters, cut the legs from the thighs and the wings from the breasts. (It will fit in your skillet more easily this way.)

Melt the butter in a heavy skillet over medium-high heat, and brown the chicken, turning it once or twice, until it's golden all over.

Pour off most of the fat, and sprinkle the chicken with the salt and just a dash of pepper. Scatter the tarragon over the chicken, crushing it a little between your fingers to release the flavor, then add the garlic and the wine.

Cover the skillet, turn the burner to low, and simmer for 30 minutes, turning the chicken at least once. Spoon a little of the pan liquid over each piece of chicken when serving.

Skillet Chicken Florentine

Olive oil

2 or 3 boneless, skinless chicken breasts

1 package (10 ounces) frozen chopped spinach, thawed

2 cloves garlic, crushed

¼ cup heavy cream

¼ cup grated Parmesan cheese

—

Yield: 3 servings, each with 5 grams of carbohydrates and 3 grams of fiber, for a total of 2 grams of usable carbs and 33 grams of protein.

Warm a little olive oil in a heavy skillet, and brown the chicken breasts over medium heat to the point where they just have a touch of gold. Remove the chicken from the skillet.

Add a couple more tablespoons of olive oil, the spinach, and the garlic, and stir for 2 to 3 minutes. Stir in the cream and cheese, and spread the mixture evenly over the bottom of the skillet. Place the chicken breasts on top, cover, turn the burner to low, and let simmer for 15 minutes.

Serve chicken breasts with the spinach on top.

Curried Chicken

4 or 5 chicken quarters, cut up and skinned

1 medium onion

1 tablespoon butter

1 rounded tablespoon curry powder

1 cup heavy cream

3 or 4 cloves of garlic, crushed

½ cup water

—

Yield: 4 generous servings, each with 6 grams of carbohydrates and 1 gram of fiber, for a total of 5 grams of usable carbs and 42 grams of protein.

Preheat the oven to 375°F.

Arrange the chicken in a shallow baking pan. Chop the onion, and scatter it over the chicken.

Melt the butter in a small, heavy skillet, and sauté the curry powder in it for a couple of minutes—just until it starts to smell good.

Mix together the cream, garlic, water, and sautéed curry powder, and pour this over the chicken. Bake it, uncovered, for 1 hour to 1 hour and 20 minutes, turning the chicken over every 20 to 30 minutes so that the sauce flavors both sides.

To serve, arrange the chicken on a platter. Take the sauce in the pan (it will look dreadful, sort of curdled up, but it will smell like heaven) and scrape it all into your blender. Blend it with a little more water or cream, if necessary, to get a nice, rich, golden sauce. Pour it over the chicken and serve.

NOTE

Ahem. Take a look at the first ingredient in this recipe—the chicken is skinned, right? Now, that's not because you can't have chicken skin on a low-carb diet, it's because cooking chicken with the skin on in a recipe like this only results in flabby, uninteresting chicken skin.

Spicy Peanut Chicken

This takes 10 minutes to put together, and only another 15 to cook. It's hot and spicy, quasi-Thai.

1 teaspoon ground cumin

½ teaspoon ground cinnamon

2 or 3 boneless, skinless chicken breasts

2 to 3 tablespoons olive or peanut oil for sautéing (I think peanut is better here)

½ smallish onion, thinly sliced

1 can (14½ ounces) diced tomatoes

2 tablespoons natural peanut butter

1 tablespoon lemon juice

2 cloves garlic, crushed

1 fresh jalapeño, cut in half and seeded

—

Yield: About 3 servings, each with 14 grams of carbohydrates and 1 gram of fiber, for a total of 13 grams of usable carbs and 26 grams of protein.

On a saucer or plate, stir the cumin and cinnamon together, then rub into both sides of chicken breasts.

Put 2 to 3 tablespoons of oil in a heavy skillet over medium heat, and add the chicken and sliced onion. Brown the chicken a bit on both sides.

While that's happening, put all the liquid and half the tomatoes from the can of tomatoes in a blender or food processor, along with the peanut butter, lemon juice, garlic, and jalapeño. (Wash your hands after handling that hot pepper, or you'll be sorry the next time you touch your eyes!) Blend or process until smooth.

Pour this rather thick sauce over the chicken (which you've turned at least once by now, right?), add the rest of the canned tomatoes, cover, turn the burner to Low, and let it sit for 10 to 15 minutes, or until the chicken is cooked through.

NOTE

Some like it hot, and some like it a little bit less so. So when you're buying your ingredients, choose a little jalapeño or a big one, depending on how hot you like your food. I use a big one, and it definitely makes this dish hot. And don't forget, there's no law against using only half a jalapeño.

Chicken and Artichoke Skillet

This is quick and easy enough for a weeknight, but elegant enough for company.

3 tablespoons butter

4 boneless, skinless chicken breasts

1 can (14 ounces) quartered artichoke hearts, drained

½ red bell pepper, cut into strips

1 medium onion, sliced

1 clove garlic, crushed

¼ cup dry white wine

1 teaspoon dried thyme

—

Yield: 4 servings, each with 8 grams of carbohydrates and 4 grams of fiber, for a total of 4 grams of usable carbs and 26 grams of protein.

Melt 2 tablespoons of butter in a heavy skillet over medium heat, and sauté the chick-en breasts until they're golden (5 to 7 minutes per side). Remove from the skillet.

Melt the remaining tablespoon of butter, and toss the artichoke hearts, pepper, onion, and garlic into the skillet. Sauté for 3 minutes or so, stirring frequently.

Pour the wine and sprinkle the thyme over the vegetables. Place the chicken breasts over the vegetables, turn the heat to medium low, cover, and simmer for 10 minutes.

Teriyaki Chicken

4 to 6 boneless, skinless chicken breasts

1 batch Teriyaki Sauce (see page 411)

—

Yield: 4 to 6 servings (depending on the number of breasts you cook), each with 2 grams of carbohydrates, a trace of fiber, and 26 grams of protein.

Put your chicken breasts in a large zipper-lock bag, and pour the teriyaki sauce over them. Stick the bag in the refrigerator, and let the breasts marinate for at least 1 hour. (More time won't hurt; if you do this in the morning, you can cook as soon as you come home at night.)

When you're ready to cook, pour off the marinade into a small saucepan. Grill or broil your chicken for 5 to 7 minutes per side, checking doneness by cutting into one breast to see if it's done. Don't overcook, or your chicken will be dry.

While your chicken is cooking, bring the marinade to a boil for a few minutes. It will then be safe to pour a little on each piece of chicken before serving.

Chicken Paprikash

Making my Paprikash with real sour cream is one of the great joys of low-carbing!

3 tablespoons butter

1 cut-up broiler-fryer

1 small onion

2 tablespoons paprika

½ cup chicken broth

1 cup sour cream

Salt or Vege-Sal and pepper

—

Yield: 4 servings, each with 7 grams of carbohydrates and 1 gram of fiber, for a total of 6 grams of usable carbs and 53 grams of protein.

Melt the butter in a heavy skillet, and brown the chicken and onions over medium-high heat.

In a separate bowl, stir the paprika into the chicken broth. Pour the mixture over the chicken.

Cover the skillet, turn the burner to low, and let it simmer for 30 to 45 minutes.

When the chicken is tender and cooked through, remove it from the skillet and put it on a serving platter. Stir the sour cream into the liquid left in the pan, and stir until smooth and well blended. Heat through, but do not let it boil, or it will curdle. Salt and pepper to taste, and serve this gravy with the chicken.

Homestyle Turkey Loaf

1 pound ground turkey

½ cup crushed pork rinds

1 rib celery, finely chopped

1 small onion, finely chopped

½ cup finely chopped apple

1½ tablespoons Worcestershire sauce

2 teaspoons poultry seasoning

1 teaspoon salt or Vege-Sal

1 egg

—

Yield: 5 servings, each with 5 grams of carbohydrates and 1 gram of fiber, for a total of 4 grams of usable carbs and 32 grams of protein.

Preheat the oven to 350°F.

Combine all the ingredients in a big bowl and—with clean hands—squeeze it together until it's very well combined.

Spray a loaf pan with nonstick cooking spray, and pack the turkey mixture into the pan. Bake for 50 minutes.

Curried Turkey Loaf

2 pounds ground turkey

1 medium onion, chopped fairly fine

2 eggs

2 cloves garlic, crushed

1 to 2 tablespoons curry powder

1 tablespoon salt or Vege-Sal

1 teaspoon pepper

—

Yield: 6 servings, each with 4 grams of carbohydrates and 1 gram of fiber, for a total of 3 grams of usable carbs and 29 grams of protein.

Preheat the oven to 350°F.

Combine all the ingredients in a big bowl and—with clean hands—squeeze it together until it's very well combined.

Spray a loaf pan with nonstick cooking spray, and pack the turkey mixture into the pan. Bake for 60 to 75 minutes.

Saltimbocca

Who says all Italian food involves pasta?

4 boneless, skinless chicken breasts

¼ pound prosciutto or good boiled ham, thinly sliced

40 leaves fresh or dry sage
(fresh is preferable)

2 tablespoons butter

2 tablespoons olive oil

½ cup dry white wine

—

Yield: 4 servings, each with 2 grams of carbohydrates, no fiber, and 37 grams of protein.

Place a chicken breast in a large, heavy, zipper-lock bag and, using a hammer, meat tenderizer, or what-have-you, pound it until it's ¼ inch thick. Repeat with the remaining chicken breasts.

Once all your chicken breasts are pounded thin, place a layer of the prosciutto on each one, scatter about 10 sage leaves over each one, and roll each breast up. Fasten with toothpicks.

Melt the butter with the olive oil in a heavy skillet over medium heat. Add the chicken rolls and sauté, turning occasionally, until golden all over.

Add the wine to the skillet, turn the burner to low, cover the skillet, and simmer for 15 minutes.

Remove the rolls to a serving plate, and cover to keep warm. Turn the burner up to High, and boil the liquid in the skillet hard for 5 minutes, to reduce. Spoon over rolls, and serve.

Key Lime Chicken

An unusual—and good!—combination of flavors.

1 cut-up broiler-fryer

½ cup lime juice

½ cup olive oil

1 tablespoon grated onion

2 teaspoons tarragon

1 teaspoon seasoned salt

¼ teaspoon pepper

—

Yield: 4 servings, each with 4 grams of carbohydrates, a trace of fiber, and 44 grams of protein.

Arrange the chicken pieces on the broiler rack, skin side down.

In a bowl, combine the lime juice, oil, onion, tarragon, salt, and pepper, and brush the chicken well with the mixture.

Broil the chicken about 8 inches from the flame for 45 to 50 minutes, turning the chicken and basting with more lime mixture every 10 minutes or so.

Chicken Taco Filling

1 pound boneless, skinless chicken breasts, or 1½ to 2 pounds chicken parts

1 cup chicken broth

2 tablespoons Taco Seasoning (see page 117)

—

Yield: 4 servings, each with 1 gram of carbohydrates, a trace of fiber, and 26 grams of protein.

If you're using chicken parts (I like to make this with leg and thigh quarters), skin them first. Put your chicken in either a large, heavy-bottomed saucepan, or in your slow cooker.

Mix together the chicken broth and the taco seasoning, and pour the mixture over the chicken. If you're cooking this on the stove top, simply cover the pot, put it over low heat, and let it simmer for about 1½ hours. If you're using a slow cooker, set the pot on Low, and leave it for 6 to 8 hours.

With either method, when the chicken is done, use two forks to tear it into largish shreds. If you've used bone-in chicken parts, this is the time to remove the bones, as well. If you've cooked this on the stove top, most of the liquid will have cooked away, but if you've used a slow cooker, there will be quite a lot of liquid, so turn the pot up to High, leave the cover off, and let the liquid cook down. Stir the chicken back into the reduced seasoning liquid, and it's ready to serve.

Deviled Chicken

4 tablespoons butter

½ cup Splenda

¼ cup spicy brown mustard

1 teaspoon salt

1 teaspoon curry powder

1 cut-up broiler-fryer

—

Yield: 4 servings, each with 5 grams of carbohydrates, a trace of fiber, and 44 grams of protein.

Preheat the oven to 375°F.

Melt the butter in a shallow roasting pan. Add the Splenda, mustard, salt, and curry powder, and stir until well combined.

Roll the chicken pieces in the butter mixture until coated, then arrange them skin side up in the pan. Bake for 1 hour.

Greek Roasted Chicken

3 to 4 pounds of chicken (whole, split in half, cut-up broiler-fryer, or cut-up parts of your choice)

¼ cup lemon juice

½ cup olive oil

½ teaspoon salt

¼ teaspoon pepper

—

Yield: 5 servings, each with less than 1 gram of carbohydrates, a bare trace of fiber, and 52 grams of protein.

Wash your chicken, and pat it dry with paper towels.

Combine the lemon juice, olive oil, salt, and pepper, and stir them together well. If you're using a whole chicken, rub it all over with some of this mixture, making sure to rub plenty inside the body cavity, as well. If you're using cut-up chicken, put it in a large zipper-lock bag, pour the marinade over it, and seal the bag.

Let the chicken marinate for at least an hour, or as long as a day.

At least 1 hour before you want to serve the chicken, pull it out of the bag. You can either grill your chicken or you can roast it in a 375°F oven for about 1 hour. Either way, cook it until the juices run clear when it's pierced to the bone.

Chicken Piccata

Meat cooked "piccata" is traditionally floured first, but with all this flavor going on, who'll miss it?

4 boneless, skinless chicken breasts

¼ cup olive oil

1 clove garlic, crushed

1 tablespoon lemon juice, or the juice of ½ lemon

½ cup dry white wine

1 tablespoon capers, chopped

3 tablespoons fresh parsley, chopped

—
Yield: 4 servings, each with 1 gram of carbohydrates, a trace of fiber, and 29 grams of protein.

Place a chicken breast in a large, heavy, zipper-lock bag and, using a hammer, meat tenderizer, or what-have-you, pound it until it's ¼ inch thick. Repeat with the remaining chicken breasts.

Heat the olive oil in a large, heavy skillet over medium-high heat. Add the chicken; if it doesn't all fit at the same time, cook it in two batches, keeping the first batch warm while the second batch is cooking. Cook the chicken until it's done through (3 to 4 minutes per side).

Remove the chicken from the pan. Add the garlic, lemon juice, white wine, and capers to the pan, stirring it all around to get the tasty little brown bits off the bottom of the pan. Boil the whole thing hard for about 1 minute, to reduce it a little.

Put the chicken back in the pan for another minute, sprinkle the parsley over it, and serve.

PORK PICCATA. Make this variation just like Chicken Piccatta, only substitute 4 good, big pork steaks, or chops, or thinly sliced pork butt (1 to 1 ½ pounds of meat total) for the chicken breasts. (Cut the bones out of the pork steaks or chops, if using, and discard.)

—
Yield: 4 servings, each with 1 gram of carbohydrates, a trace of fiber, and 26 grams of protein.

Lemon-Pepper Chicken and Gravy

1 cut-up broiler-fryer

1¼ teaspoons lemon pepper

1¼ teaspoons onion powder

1 teaspoon salt

¼ cup chicken broth

½ cup heavy cream

1½ teaspoons spicy brown or Dijon mustard

—

Yield: 4 servings, each with 2 grams of carbohydrates, a trace of fiber, and 44 grams of protein.

Preheat the oven to 375°F.

Sprinkle the chicken pieces with 1 teaspoon of lemon pepper, 1 teaspoon of onion powder, and the salt. Arrange in a roasting pan, and roast, basting once or twice, for about 1 hour or until the juices run clear when the chicken is pierced.

Remove the chicken from the roasting pan and skim off the excess fat, leaving just the brown drippings. Place the roasting pan over a low burner, add the chicken broth to the pan, and stir, scraping up the tasty brown bits off the bottom of the pan. When the broth is simmering, add the cream, the rest of the lemon pepper and onion powder, and the mustard. Stir well, heat through, and pour over the chicken.

Thai-ish Chicken Basil Stir-Fry

If all you've had are Chinese stir-fries, you'll find this an interesting change.

2 tablespoons Thai fish sauce (nam pla)

2 tablespoons soy sauce

1 teaspoon Splenda

¼ teaspoon guar or xanthan

2 teaspoons dried basil

1½ teaspoons red pepper flakes

Peanut, canola, or coconut oil

2 cloves garlic, crushed

3 boneless, skinless chicken breasts cut into ½-inch cubes

1 small onion, sliced

1½ cups frozen, crosscut green beans, thawed

—

Yield: 3 servings, each with 13 grams of carbohydrates and 3 grams of fiber, for a total of 10 grams of usable carbs and 31 grams of protein.

Combine the fish sauce, soy sauce, Splenda, and guar in a blender. Blend for several seconds, then turn off the blender and add the basil and red pepper flakes, and set aside.

Heat a few tablespoons of oil in a wok or heavy skillet over high heat. When the oil is hot, add the garlic, chicken, and onion, and stir-fry for 3 to 4 minutes. Add the green beans, and continue to stir-fry until the chicken is done through.

Stir the blended seasoning mixture into the stir-fry, turn the burner to medium, cover, and let it simmer for 2 to 3 minutes (the beans should be tender-crisp).

Sautéed Sesame Chicken Breasts

Try serving this with a salad, a broccoli dish, or both.

4 boneless, skinless chicken breasts

¼ cup sesame seeds

Salt

3 tablespoons peanut oil

—

Yield: 4 servings, each with 2 grams of carbohydrates and 1 gram of fiber, for a total of 1 gram of usable carbs and 30 grams of protein.

Place a chicken breast in a large, heavy, zipper-lock bag and, using a hammer, meat tenderizer, or what-have-you, pound it until it's ¼ inch thick. Repeat with the remaining chicken breasts.

Sprinkle each side of each breast evenly with ½ tablespoon of sesame seeds, and lightly salt.

Heat the peanut oil in a heavy skillet over medium heat. Add the chicken breasts and sauté for about 5 minutes each side, or until lightly golden. (You may have to do this in two batches; keep the first batch warm on an oven-proof plate in the oven, on its lowest temperature setting.) Serve.

Stewed Chicken with Moroccan Seasonings

This is almost a Moroccan "tangine," but all the recipes I've seen call for some sort of starch. So I ditched the starch and just kept the seasonings, which are exotic and delicious.

¼ cup olive oil

3½ to 4 pounds chicken, cut up

1 medium onion, thinly sliced

2 cloves garlic, crushed

¾ cup chicken broth

½ teaspoon ground coriander

½ teaspoon ground cinnamon

½ teaspoon paprika

½ teaspoon ground cumin

1 teaspoon ground ginger

½ teaspoon pepper

¼ teaspoon cayenne

1 tablespoon Splenda

1 tablespoon tomato paste

1 teaspoon salt or Vege-Sal

—
Yield: 4 generous servings, each with 6 grams of carbohydrates and 1 gram of fiber, for a total of 5 grams of usable carbs and 58 grams of protein.

Heat the oil in a Dutch oven over medium heat, and brown the chicken in the oil.

When the chicken is golden all over, remove it from the Dutch oven, and pour off the fat. Put the chicken back in the Dutch oven, and scatter the onion and garlic over it.

Combine the garlic, broth, coriander, cinnamon, paprika, cumin, ginger, pepper, cayenne, Splenda, tomato paste, and salt, and whisk together well. Pour over the chicken, cover the Dutch oven, and turn the burner to low. Let the whole thing simmer for a good 45 minutes.

Uncover the chicken and let it simmer for another 15 minutes or so, to let the juices concentrate a bit. Serve each piece of chicken with some of the onion and juices spooned over it.

CHAPTER 7

Beef, Pork, and Lamb

There seems to be no end to the ways we can use beef—by itself, in casseroles, and in sandwiches, sauces, and pizzas, beef is a delicious way to get plenty of protein for no carbs at all. This chapter gives you some low-carb editions of high-carb favorites, as well as showing you some ways to use beef that you may never have even considered before. So read on.

Bleu Burger

1 hamburger patty

1 tablespoon crumbled blue cheese

1 teaspoon finely minced sweet red onion

—

Yield: 1 serving, with only a trace of carbohydrates, no fiber, and 27 grams of protein.

Cook your burger by your preferred method. When it's almost done to your liking, top with the bleu cheese and let it melt. Remove from the heat, put it on plate, and top with onion.

Smothered Burgers

Mmmmushrooms and onions!

4 hamburger patties

2 tablespoons butter or olive oil

½ cup sliced onion

½ cup sliced mushrooms

Dash of Worcestershire sauce

—

Yield: 4 servings, each with just 2 grams of carbohydrates, at least a trace of fiber, and 27 grams of protein.

Cook your burgers by your preferred method. While the burgers are cooking, melt the butter or heat the oil in a small, heavy skillet over medium-high heat. Add the onion and mushrooms, and sauté until the onions are translucent. Add a dash of Worcestershire sauce, stir, and spoon over burgers.

Ground Beef "Helper"

When your family starts agitating for the "normal" food of yore, whip up this recipe.

1 pound lean ground beef or ground turkey

½ cup chopped green pepper

½ cup chopped onion

½ cup diced celery

2 cans (8 ounces each) tomato sauce

2 cloves garlic, crushed; 1 teaspoon minced garlic; or ½ teaspoon garlic powder

½ teaspoon Italian seasoning

2 cups shredded Cheddar or Monterey Jack cheese

1 box (about 1 ¾ ounces) low-carb pasta

⅓ cup water

Salt and pepper to taste

—

Yield: 6 servings, each with 11 grams of carbohydrates and 2 grams of fiber, for a total of 9 grams of usable carbs and 36 grams of protein.

In a large, oven-safe skillet, brown the meat with the pepper, onion, and celery. Drain off the grease.

Add the tomato sauce, garlic, seasoning, 1 cup of the cheese, pasta, water, and salt and pepper to taste. Cover and simmer over low heat for 10 minutes. Turn on broiler to preheat during last the few minutes of cooking time.

Stir well. Spread the remaining 1 cup of cheese over the top, and broil until the cheese starts to brown.

Mexican Meatballs

Marilee Wellersdick sends this easy, South-of-the-Border skillet meal.

1 pound ground beef or ground turkey

2 eggs

1 medium onion, finely chopped

3 cloves garlic, minced

2 teaspoons ground coriander

½ teaspoon salt

2 tablespoons oil

1 can (14½ ounces) cut or crushed tomatoes

1 can (8 ounces) tomato sauce

1 tablespoon chili powder

½ teaspoon ground cumin

—
Yield: 4 servings, each with 15 grams of carbohydrates and 3 grams of fiber, for a total of 12 grams of usable carbs and 24 grams of protein.

Mix together the ground beef, eggs, half of the onion, two-thirds of the garlic, coriander, and salt. Shape the mixture into 2-inch balls.

Heat the oil in a large skillet. Add the meatballs and brown them. Add the tomatoes, tomato sauce, the remaining half of the onion, the remaining third of the garlic, chili powder, and cumin to the skillet. Cover and simmer over medium-low heat for 45 minutes.

Sloppy José

1 pound ground beef

1 cup salsa (mild, medium, or hot, as you prefer)

1 cup shredded Mexican-style cheese

—

Yield: About 4 servings, each with 4 grams of carbohydrates and 1 gram of fiber, for a total of 3 grams of usable carbs and 27 grams of protein.

In a large skillet, crumble and brown the ground beef, and drain off the fat.

Stir in the salsa and cheese, and heat until the cheese is melted.

MEGA SLOPPY JOSÉ. Try adding another ½ cup salsa and another ½ cup cheese.

—

Yield: 4 servings, each with 6 grams of carbohydrates and 2 grams of fiber, for a total of 4 grams of usable carbs and 30 grams of protein.

All-Meat Chili

2 pounds ground beef

1 cup chopped onion

3 cloves garlic, crushed

1 can (14½ ounces) tomatoes with green chilies

1 can (4 ounces) plain tomato sauce

4 teaspoons ground cumin

2 teaspoons dried oregano

2 teaspoons unsweetened cocoa powder

1 teaspoon paprika

—

Yield: 6 servings, each with 7 grams of carbohydrates and 2 grams of fiber, for a total of 5 grams of usable carbs and 27 grams of protein.

Brown and crumble the beef in a heavy skillet over medium-high heat. Pour off the grease, and add the onion, garlic, tomatoes, tomato sauce, cumin, oregano, cocoa, and paprika. Stir to combine.

Turn the burner to low, cover, and simmer for 30 minutes. Uncover and simmer for another 15 to 20 minutes, or until the chili thickens a bit. Serve with grated cheese, sour cream, chopped raw onion, or other low-carb toppings.

Beef Taco Filling

1 pound ground beef

2 tablespoons Taco Seasoning (see page 117)

¼ cup water

—

Yield: 4 servings, each with less than 1 gram of carbohydrates, no fiber, and 19 grams of protein.

Brown and crumble the ground beef in a heavy skillet over medium-high heat.

When the meat is cooked through, drain the grease and stir in the seasoning and water. Let it simmer for about 5 minutes, and serve.

Reuben Casserole

Another great recipe from Vicki Cash. Thanks, Vicki!

4 small summer squash or zucchini

2 tablespoons water

1 can (27 ounces) sauerkraut, drained

1 tablespoon caraway seeds

2 tablespoons Dijon mustard

8 ounces shaved corned beef or pastrami

4 ounces grated Swiss cheese

—

Yield: 4 servings, each with 16 grams of carbohydrates and 8 grams of fiber, for a total of 8 grams of usable carbs and 21 grams of protein.

Slice the squash into bite-size pieces. Place the pieces in a 2-quart microwave-safe casserole, and add the water. Cover and microwave on High for 3 minutes.

Add the sauerkraut, caraway seeds, mustard, and meat, mixing well. Cover and microwave on High for 6 minutes, stirring halfway through.

Stir in the cheese, and microwave for 3 to 5 more minutes, or until the cheese is melted.

Steakhouse Steak

Ever wonder why steak is better at a steakhouse than it is at home? Part of it is that the best grades of meat are reserved for the restaurants, but it's also the method: quick grilling, at very high heat, very close to the flame. Try it at home, with this recipe.

Olive oil

1½ to 2 pounds well-marbled steak (sirloin, rib eye, or the like), 1 to 1½ inches thick

—

Yield: The number of servings will depend on the size of your steak, but what you really need to know is that there are no carbs here at all.

Rub a couple of teaspoons of olive oil on either side of the steak.

Arrange your broiler so you can get the steak so close that it's almost, but not quite, touching the broiling element. (I have to put my broiler pan on top of a skillet turned upside down to do this.) Turn the broiler to high, and get that steak in there. Leave the oven door open—this is crucial. For a 1-inch-thick steak, set the oven timer for 5 to 5½ minutes; for a 1½-inch-thick steak, you can go up to 6 minutes.

When the timer beeps, quickly flip the steak, and set the timer again. Check at this point to see if your time seems right. If you like your steak a lot rarer or more well-done than I do, or if you have a different brand of broiler, you may need to adjust how long you broil the second side for.

When the timer goes off again, get that steak out of there quickly, put it on a serving plate, and season it any way you like.

Southwestern Steak

I adore steak, I adore guacamole, and the combination is fantastic.

Olive oil

1½ to 2 pounds well-marbled steak (sirloin, rib eye, or the like), 1 to 1½ inches thick

Guacamole (see page 24)

Salt and pepper

—

Yield: The number of servings will depend on the size of your steak, but the guacamole will add 4 grams of carbohydrates and 1 gram of fiber, for a total of 3 grams of usable carbs. You'll also get 275 milligrams of potassium.

Prepare the Steakhouse Steak (see page 92) to your preferred degree of doneness. Spread each serving of steak with a heaping tablespoon of guacamole, and salt and pepper to taste.

Cajun Steak

2 to 3 teaspoons Cajun Seasoning

1 pound sirloin steak, 1 inch thick

—

Yield: 3 or 4 servings; the Cajun seasoning adds a bare trace of carbohydrates to each.

Simply sprinkle Cajun seasoning over both sides of your steak. Then either pan-broil it (cook in on a very hot, ungreased, heavy skillet) or cook it on a stove top grill over maximum heat. Either way, cook it just 6½ minutes per side.

Steak Vinaigrette

You don't have to make a batch of homemade vinaigrette every time you want a steak; store-bought will work just as well here.

Steak, in your preferred cut and quantity

½ cup vinaigrette dressing for each pound of steak

—

Yield: assume 1 pound of steak is 2 servings, each with about 1 gram of carbohydrates, maximum, no fiber, and 33 grams of protein.

Put your steak in a 1-quart zipper-lock bag, and pour the vinaigrette dressing over it. Let the steak marinate for at least 15 minutes, or leave it all day, if you have the time.

When you're ready to cook your steak, remove it from the bag, discard the marinade, and broil or grill it, as you prefer (see page 92).

Beef Gravy

Faced with leftover roast beef, and no gravy, I came up with this, and it's as good as any beef gravy I've ever had. If you have any nice, brown beef juices from your roast, they can only improve it further, but be sure to skim off the fat before adding them, as it will ruin the texture.

1 can (14½ ounces) beef broth

2 tablespoons dry red wine

1 teaspoon liquid beef bouillon concentrate

1 tablespoon finely minced onion

1 small clove garlic, crushed

¾ teaspoon guar or xanthan

⅓ cup heavy cream

¼ teaspoon Gravy Master or similar gravy seasoning/coloring liquid

Salt and pepper

—

Yield: Makes 8 servings of 2 tablespoons, each with less than 2 grams of carbohydrates and 1 gram of fiber, for a total of just under 1 gram of usable carbs and 3 grams of protein.

In a heavy saucepan, combine the broth, wine, bouillon concentrate, onion, and garlic. Bring this to a boil over medium heat, and let it boil until reduced to one-third the original volume. (This will take at least 15 to 20 minutes.)

When the mixture is reduced, pour it into a blender (if you're not sure your blender will take the heat, let it cool for 5 to 10 minutes first), turn it on, and add the guar. Blend for 15 seconds or so. Pour it back into the saucepan, turn the heat back on to low, and whisk in the cream and the gravy seasoning liquid. Salt and pepper to taste, heat through, and serve.

Italian Herb Pork Chops

For each serving you'll need:

1 clove garlic, crushed

1 pork chop, 1 inch thick

½ teaspoon dried, powdered sage

½ teaspoon dried, powdered rosemary

Salt or Vege-Sal

2 tablespoons dry white wine

—

Yield: 1 serving, with 2 grams of carbohydrates, a trace of fiber, and about 23 grams of protein.

Rub the crushed garlic into both sides of your pork chop.

In a bowl, mix the sage and rosemary together, and sprinkle this evenly over both sides of the pork chop, as well. Sprinkle lightly with the salt.

Place the chops in a heavy skillet (if you're feeding several people, you may well need two skillets), and add water just up to the top edge of the pork chop. Cover the skillet, turn the burner to low, and let the chop simmer for about 1 hour, or until the water has all evaporated.

Once the water is gone, the chop will start to brown. Turn it once or twice to get it browned on both sides. (The pork chop will be very tender, so use a spatula and be careful, but if it breaks a little, it will still taste great.)

Remove the porkchop to a serving platter, and pour the wine into the skillet. Turn up the burner to medium-high, and stir the wine around, scraping up the stuck-on brown bits from the pan. Bring this to a boil, and let it boil hard for a minute or two to reduce it just a little. Pour this sauce over the pork chop, and serve.

Looed Pork

This is a great way to add a lot of flavor to the usually bland boneless pork loin.

1½ pounds boneless pork loin, sliced about 1½ inch thick

1 batch Looing Sauce (see page 123)

Scallions, sliced

Toasted sesame oil

—

Yield: 4 generous servings with no more than 1 gram of carbohydrates, no fiber, and 35 grams of protein.

Put the pork in a slow cooker, pour the looing sauce over it, cover the cooker, and set it to Low. Forget about it for 8 to 9 hours.

At dinnertime, remove the pieces of pork from the looing sauce. Put each piece on a serving plate, scatter a few sliced scallions over each serving, and top with a few drops of toasted sesame oil.

Mu Shu Pork

I hear from lots of people that they miss Chinese food, so here's a Chinese restaurant favorite, de-carbed. Low-carb tortillas stand in here for mu shu pancakes, and they work fine. If you want to de-carb this even further, just eat it with a fork and forget the tortillas.

3 eggs, beaten

Peanut oil

½ cup slivered mushrooms

8 ounces boneless pork loin, sliced across the grain and then cut into matchsticks

1 cup shredded napa cabbage

3 scallions, sliced

1 cup bean sprouts

3 tablespoons soy sauce

2 tablespoons dry sherry

4 low-carb tortillas

Hoisin Sauce (see page 116)

—

Yield: 2 servings, each with 11 grams of carbohydrates and 3 grams of fiber, for a total of 8 grams of usable carbs and 27 grams of protein (Analysis does not include low-carb tortillas or hoisin sauce.)

First, in a wok or heavy skillet over high heat, scramble the eggs in a few tablespoons of the peanut oil until they're set but still moist. Remove and set aside.

Wipe the wok out if there's much egg clinging to it. Add another ¼ cup or so of peanut oil, and heat. Add the pork, and stir-fry until it's mostly done. Add the cabbage, scallions, and sprouts, and stir-fry for 3 to 4 minutes. Add the eggs back into the wok, and stir them in, breaking them into small pieces. Now add the soy sauce and sherry, and stir.

To serve, take a warmed, low-carb tortilla, and smear about 2 teaspoons of hoisin sauce on it. Put about a quarter of the stir-fry mixture on the tortilla, and wrap it up.

NOTE

Make sure you have everything cut up and ready to go before you cook a thing, and this recipe will be a breeze.

Robinsky's Cabbage & Sausage

Robin Wilkins says this makes a great one-plate meal. Just make sure you read the labels on the kielbasa carefully, as they vary widely in carb count.

2 to 3 tablespoons butter

1 medium onion, chopped

1 pound Polska Kielbasa or similar low-carb sausage, sliced

1 head cabbage, chopped

—

Yield: 3 servings. The carb content of this depends completely on the sausage used. Using a low-carb sausage, each serving has 8 grams of carbohydrates and 1 gram of fiber, for a total of 7 grams of usable carbs and 21 grams of protein.

Divide the butter between two skillets. Sauté the onion and sausage in one and sauté the cabbage in the other. The cabbage will overwhelm your frying pan at first, but it will reduce in volume as it fries.

When cooked to the texture you like (I like mine tender-crisp), combine the contents of both skillets, and toss.

Mediterranean Leg of Lamb

Lamb makes a wonderful Sunday dinner roast. If you don't want to roast a whole leg of lamb at once because it's a lot of meat, ask the butcher to cut one leg into two roasts. Make half now, and freeze the other half for another day.

Leg of lamb, with or without the bone in.

1 cup dry red wine

1 cup olive oil

5 cloves garlic, crushed

3 tablespoons lemon juice

1 tablespoon dried rosemary

1 tablespoon dried oregano

—

Yield: 3 servings per pound, each with no carbohydrates or fiber to speak of, and about 21 grams of protein. (This sounds low, I know, but remember: Part of that weight is bone.)

NOTE

Make Lamb Gravy (see page 99) to go with your roast lamb, and serve it with some Cauliflower Rice (see page 61).

Place your leg of lamb in a pan large enough to hold it.

Combine the wine, ½ cup of the olive oil, 3 cloves of the garlic, and the lemon juice, rosemary, and oregano. Pour this marinade over the lamb, and let the lamb sit in it for at least 5 to 6 hours, turning it from time to time.

When the time comes to cook your lamb, preheat the oven to 425°F. Remove the meat from the marinade and place it on a rack in a roasting pan. Leave the rosemary needles and bits of oregano clinging to it.

Combine the remaining olive oil and cloves of garlic, and spoon this mixture over the lamb, coating the whole leg. Position the leg with the fat side up and insert a meat thermometer deep into the center of the thickest part of the meat, but don't let it touch the bone.

When the oven is up to temperature, put your roast in and set the timer for 10 minutes. After 10 minutes, turn the oven down to 350°F, and roast for about 30 minutes per pound of meat, or until the meat thermometer registers 170° to 180°F. Remove the lamb from the oven, and let it sit for 15 to 20 minutes before carving.

Lamb Gravy

Drippings from Mediterranean Leg of Lamb
(see page 98)

1 cup chicken broth

¾ teaspoon guar or xanthan

Salt and pepper to taste

—

Yield: The only carbohydrates in this gravy will be some fiber from the guar or xanthan, plus maybe 1 gram per serving from the herbs and wine.

NOTE

The easiest way to skim drippings is to pour them into a large, heavy, zipper-lock bag. Seal the bag, and tip it so one corner points down over the roasting pan. Let it hang this way for a minute or so, until you see the fat float to the top and the good, flavorful, dark-colored pan juices at the bottom. Snip a tiny triangle off the bottom corner of the bag, and let the juices run out. Grab the corner of the bag to stop the flow before the fat runs into the pan, and throw the bag and the grease away.

Skim the fat off of the drippings from the roast. (Fat will ruin the texture of your gravy.)

Pour ½ cup of the chicken broth into the roasting pan with the skimmed drippings, and stir it around, scraping up the yummy browned bits from the rack and the bottom of the pan. When most of the stuck-on stuff is dissolved into the broth, put the roasting pan over medium-high heat.

Put the rest of the chicken broth in a blender with the guar or xanthan, and run the blender for a few seconds to dissolve all of the thickener. Pour the thickened broth into the roasting pan, and stir until all the gravy is thickened. (If it gets too thick, add a little more chicken broth; if it's not quite thick enough, let it simmer for a few minutes to cook down.)

Salt and pepper the gravy to taste, and serve with the leg of lamb.

CHAPTER 8

Main Dish Salads

In the first edition of this book, I wrote: "I think main dish salads are one of the very best things for a low-carber to eat, because they offer infinite variety. Of course, they contain enough vegetables that you probably won't want to eat much else in the way of carbohydrates at that particular meal, but with all the flavor and eye appeal these salads offer, who needs anything else?"

Dilled Chicken Salad

1½ cups cooked chicken, diced

1 large rib celery, diced

½ green pepper, diced

¼ medium, sweet red onion, diced

3 tablespoons mayonnaise

3 tablespoons sour cream

1 teaspoon dried dill weed

Salt

—

Yield: 2 servings, each with 5 grams of carbohydrates and 1 gram of fiber, for a total of 4 grams of usable carbs and 24 grams of protein.

Combine the chicken, celery, pepper, and onion in a bowl.

In a separate bowl, mix together the mayonnaise, sour cream, and dill. Pour the mixture over the chicken and veggies, toss, salt to taste, and serve.

NOTE

This is wonderful when made with leftover turkey, too.

Chicken Caesar Salad

1 boneless, skinless chicken breast

2 to 3 cups romaine lettuce, washed, dried, and broken up

2 tablespoons Caesar Dressing (bottled, or see page 113)

2 tablespoons Parmesan cheese, in thin slivers or grated

—

Yield: 1 serving, with 5 grams of carbohydrates and 2 grams of fiber, for a total of 3 grams of usable carbs and 26 grams of protein.

Grill the chicken breast. (I do mine in an electric tabletop grill for about 5 minutes, but you could sauté it, if you prefer.)

While the chicken cooks, put the lettuce in a bowl, pour the dressing over it, and toss well. Pile it on your serving plate.

Slice the cooked chicken breast into thin strips, and pile it on top of the lettuce. Scatter the Parmesan on top, and dig in.

SHRIMP CAESAR SALAD. Make this just like Chicken Caesar Salad (above), but substitute 10 to 12 good-size cooked shrimp for the chicken breast. Frozen, precooked, shelled shrimp are handy for this because they thaw quickly, especially if you put them in a zipper-lock baggie and set them in warm tap water for a few minutes.

—

Yield: 5 grams of carbohydrates and 2 grams of fiber, for a total of 3 grams of usable carbs and 30 grams of protein.

Asian Chicken Salad

This is an wonderful salad, different from any I've ever tried. Do use rice vinegar instead of another kind, and napa cabbage instead of regular. They may seem like small distinctions, but they make all the difference.

2 tablespoons oil

½ cup walnuts, chopped

4 boneless, skinless chicken breasts

3 cups thinly sliced bok choy

3 cups thinly sliced napa cabbage

¼ cup grated carrots

1 cucumber, thinly sliced

½ cup sliced scallions

½ cup chopped fresh cilantro

⅓ cup soy sauce

¼ cup rice vinegar

1 tablespoon lime juice

2 tablespoons Splenda

3 cloves garlic, crushed

½ teaspoon red pepper flakes (or to taste)

—
Yield: 4 generous servings, each with 15 grams of carbohydrates and 4 grams of fiber, for a total of 11 grams of usable carbs and 36 grams of protein.

Put the oil in a heavy skillet over medium heat and toast the walnuts, stirring for about 4 to 5 minutes or until they're brown and crisp. Set aside.

Grill your chicken breasts, and slice them into strips; I use my electric tabletop grill, but you can use whatever method you prefer.

Combine the bok choy, cabbage, carrots, cucumber, scallions, and cilantro in a big bowl.

In a separate bowl, combine the soy sauce, rice vinegar, lime juice, Splenda, garlic, and red pepper flakes. Pour about two-thirds of this dressing over the salad, and toss well, coating all the vegetables.

Heap the salad onto four serving plates, top each with a sliced chicken breast, and drizzle the rest of the dressing over them. Sprinkle with chopped walnuts, and serve.

NOTE

We generally only have 2 people to eat all this salad, so I set half of the vegetable mixture aside in a container in the refrigerator. Don't put dressing on the half you plan to reserve, just put the dry, shredded vegetables in a container in the fridge, save half of your dressing to go with it, and reserve some of the walnuts, as well. This is wonderful to have on hand for a quick, gourmet lunch—just grill a chicken breast, toss the salad with the dressing, and presto, lunch is served.

Taco Salad

A great summer supper. The wild card in this recipe is the ranch dressing—different brands vary tremendously in carb count. Choose a really, really low-carb one, and you'll drop the carb count below what's listed here.

2 quarts romaine or iceberg lettuce, washed, dried, and broken up

1 cup diced green pepper

½ medium cucumber, sliced

1 medium tomato, sliced into thin wedges, or 15 cherry tomatoes, halved

½ cup diced sweet red onion

½ ripe avocado, peeled, seeded, and cut into small chunks

½ cup cilantro, chopped (optional)

1 can (4 ounces) sliced black olives, drained (optional)

⅔ cup salsa plus additional for topping

½ cup ranch dressing

1 batch Chicken or Beef Taco Filling (see pages 80 and 91)

1 cup shredded Cheddar or Monterey Jack cheese

Sour cream

—

Yield: 6 servings, each with 12 grams of carbohydrates and 4 grams of fiber, for a total of 8 grams of usable carbs and 22 grams of protein.

Put the lettuce, pepper, cucumber, tomato, onion, avocado, cilantro (if using), and olives (if using) in a large salad bowl.

Stir together the ⅔ cup of salsa and the ranch dressing, pour it over the salad, and toss.

Divide the salad between the serving plates, and top each one with the taco filling and shredded cheese. Put the salsa and sour cream on the table, so folks can add their own.

Sesame Asparagus Salad

This is from Jennifer Eloff's wonderful cookbook Splendid Low-Carbing. Jen, of sweety.com, says it's simple, yet it has an eye-catching presentation.

1 pound fresh asparagus

5 cups water

4 teaspoons soy sauce

2 teaspoons sesame or olive oil

1 tablespoon sesame seeds

—

Yield: 6 servings, each with 2 grams of carbohydrates and 1 gram of fiber, for a total of 1 gram of usable carbs and 1 gram of protein.

Break off the tough ends of the asparagus by bending each stalk back until it snaps.

Bring the water to a boil in a large saucepan, and drop the asparagus stalks into the rapidly boiling water. Parboil for 5 minutes, drain immediately, and rinse in cold water. Pat dry with paper towels.

Combine the soy sauce and oil in a small bowl. Lay the asparagus stalks in a casserole, and toss with the soy sauce mixture.

Sprinkle with the sesame seeds, and chill in the refrigerator for an hour or two before serving.

Coleslaw

This is my standard coleslaw recipe, and it always draws compliments. The tiny bit of onion really sparks the flavor.

1 head green cabbage

¼ sweet red onion

Coleslaw Dressing (see page 113)

—

Yield: 10 servings, each with 1 gram of carbohydrates, a trace of fiber, and 1 gram of protein.

Using a food processor's slicing blade or a sharp knife, reduce your cabbage to little bitty shreds, and put those shreds in a great big bowl.

Mince the onion really fine, and put that in the bowl, too.

Pour on the dressing, and toss well.

NOTE

Just get invited to a picnic, and short on time for making something that'll feed a crowd? This recipe makes a veritable bucketful, and it's a wonderful side dish to almost any plain meat, including chops and chicken. If you like, you could even use bagged coleslaw from the grocery store and just add my dressing; I promise not to tell!

Coleslaw for Company

The colors in this slaw are so intense, it's almost too beautiful to eat.

1 head red cabbage

1 small carrot, shredded

¼ sweet red onion, finely minced

Coleslaw Dressing (see page 113)

—

Yield: 10 servings, each with 2 grams of carbohydrates, a trace of fiber, and 1 gram of protein.

Using a food processor's slicing blade or a sharp knife, shred your cabbage and put it in a big bowl.

Add the carrot and onion, and toss with the dressing. Admire, and enjoy.

Coleslaw Italiano

My sister makes this recipe, and it's quite good.

4 cups shredded cabbage

½ cup Italian Vinaigrette Dressing (see page 107 or use bottled)

—

Yield: 8 servings, each with 3 grams of carbohydrates and 1 gram of fiber, for a total of 2 grams of usable carbs and 1 gram of protein.

Toss the cabbage with the Italian dressing, and serve.

Mayonnaise

If you have a blender, making your own sugar-free mayonnaise is a snap. If you're on a paleo diet or an antiyeast diet, use 3 tablespoons of lemon juice and omit the vinegar. (Don't feel, by the way, that the presence of this recipe means that jarred mayonnaise is off-limits for most low-carbers; it isn't. I just thought you ought to know how easy and good it is when made from scratch.)

1 egg

1 teaspoon dry mustard

1 teaspoon salt

Dash of Tabasco

1½ tablespoons vinegar

1½ tablespoons lemon juice

½ to ⅔ cup olive or other vegetable oil

—
Yield: a little over 1 cup, with just a trace of carbohydrates, fiber, and protein—it's mostly healthy fat!

Place the egg, mustard, salt, Tabasco, vinegar, and lemon juice in the blender. Have the oil ready in a measuring cup.

Turn on the blender, and let it run for a second. With the blender running, pour in oil in a very thin stream—no thicker than a pencil lead. The mayonnaise will start to thicken before your eyes. When it gets thick enough that the "whirlpool" disappears and oil starts to collect on top, stop adding oil and turn off the blender.

Store your mayo in a tightly covered jar in the refrigerator, and keep in mind that homemade mayonnaise does not have the shelf life that the commercial kind does.

DRESSINGS

These dressings are a great place to use homemade mayonnaise, although jarred is fine, too. Some of these recipes will give you leftovers that you should store in your refrigerator, but not for as long as you would a commercial dressing. And my general rule is this: 6 servings is about what I'd put on a large, family-size salad. So if you see "12 servings," figure that you can get two salads out of it if you're a family of 6, more if you have a smaller family.

French Vinaigrette Dressing

No, this is not that sweet, tomatoey stuff that somehow has gotten the name "French dressing." No Frenchman would eat that stuff on a bet! This is a classic vinaigrette dressing.

½ **teaspoon salt**

¼ **teaspoon pepper**

¼ to⅓ **cup wine vinegar**

½ **teaspoon Dijon mustard**

¾ **cup extra-virgin olive oil**

—

Yield: 12 servings, each with only a trace of carbohydrates, fiber, and protein.

Put all the ingredients in a container with a tight lid, and shake well. Shake again before pouring over salad and tossing.

> **NOTE**
>
> The French Vinaigrette and Italian Vinaigrette Dressing recipes make approximately enough for two big, family-size salads, but feel free to double them and keep them in the fridge.

Italian Vinaigrette Dressing

Add a little zip to the French Vinaigrette, and you've got Italian Vinaigrette.

⅓ cup wine vinegar

2 cloves garlic, crushed

½ teaspoon oregano

¼ teaspoon basil

1 or 2 drops Tabasco

⅔ cup extra-virgin olive oil

Put all the ingredients in a container with a tight-fitting lid, and shake well.

—
Yield: 12 servings, each with 1 gram of carbohydrates, a trace of fiber, and a trace of protein.

CREAMY ITALIAN DRESSING. This is a simple variation on the Italian Vinaigrette. Just add 2 tablespoons of mayonnaise to the Italian Vinaigrette Dressing and whisk until smooth.

—
Yield: 12 servings, each with 1 gram of carbohydrates, a trace of fiber, and a trace of protein.

Greek Lemon Dressing

The use of lemon juice in place of vinegar in salad dressings is distinctively Greek.

¾ cup extra-virgin olive oil

¼ cup lemon juice

2 tablespoons dried oregano, crushed

1 clove garlic, crushed

Salt and pepper

Put all the ingredients in a container with a tight-fitting lid, and shake well.

NOTE

This is best made at least a few hours in advance, but don't try to double the recipe and keep it around. Lemon juice just doesn't hold its freshness the way vinegar does.

—
Yield: 12 servings, each with 1 gram of carbohydrates, a trace of fiber, and a trace of protein.

Doreen's Dressing

My friend Doreen made this up, and told me about it when I told her I was writing a cookbook. So I tried it and discovered that it's simple and wonderful.

½ cup mayonnaise

3 tablespoons balsamic vinegar

1 clove garlic, crushed

—

Yield: 6 servings, each with 1 gram of carbohydrates, a trace of fiber, and a trace of protein.

Simply combine all ingredients, and store in container with a tight-fitting lid.

Ranch Dressing

1 cup mayonnaise

1 cup buttermilk

2 tablespoons finely chopped green onions

¼ teaspoon onion powder

2 tablespoons minced fresh parsley

1 clove garlic, crushed

¼ teaspoon paprika

⅛ teaspoon cayenne powder or a few drops of Tabasco

¼ teaspoon salt

¼ teaspoon black pepper

—

Yield: about 24 servings, each with 1 gram of carbohydrates, a trace of fiber, and 1 gram of protein.

Combine all ingredients well, and store in the refrigerator, in a container with a tight-fitting lid.

Tangy "Honey" Mustard Dressing

You know that honey, despite being "natural," is pure sugar, right? Make this instead.

¼ cup canola oil

2 tablespoons apple cider vinegar

2 tablespoons spicy brown or Dijon mustard

1 tablespoon plus 2 teaspoons Splenda

⅛ teaspoon pepper

⅛ teaspoon salt

—

Yield: 6 servings, each with 1 gram of carbohydrates, a trace of fiber, and a trace of protein.

Combine all ingredients, and store in a container with a tight-fitting lid.

NOTE

This makes a little over ½ cup, or just enough for one big salad, but feel free to double, or even quadruple, this recipe.

Mellow "Honey" Mustard Dressing

1¼ cup mayonnaise

¼ cup spicy brown mustard

⅓ cup Splenda

4 tablespoons water

1 teaspoon salt

—

Yield: 12 servings, each with 1 gram of carbohydrates, a trace of fiber, and 1 gram of protein.

Combine all ingredients, and store in the refrigerator, in a container with a tight-fitting lid.

Raspberry Vinegar

Commercial raspberry vinegar has as much as 4 grams of carbohydrates per tablespoon, so keep a batch of this on hand.

½ cup white vinegar

¼ teaspoon raspberry cake flavoring (this is a highly concentrated oil in a teeny little bottle)

3 tablespoons Splenda

Just combine these ingredients, and store in a container with a tight-fitting lid.

—
Yield: about ½ cup, with 11.5 grams of carbohydrates in the whole batch or 1.5 grams of carbohydrates per tablespoon, no fiber, and no protein.

Raspberry Vinaigrette Dressing

Sweet and tangy, raspberry vinaigrette is a favorite you'll get to enjoy more often once you're making your own low-carb variety.

¼ cup Raspberry Vinegar (see above)

¼ cup canola or other bland oil

3 tablespoons plus 1 teaspoon mayonnaise

1 teaspoon spicy brown or Dijon mustard

Pinch salt and pepper

Blend all the ingredients, and store in the refrigerator, in a container with a tight-fitting lid.

—
Yield: 6 servings, each with a trace of carbohydrates, fiber, and protein.

Parmesan Peppercorn Dressing

2 tablespoons olive oil

3 tablespoons mayonnaise

2 tablespoons wine vinegar

3 tablespoons grated Parmesan cheese

1 teaspoon freshly ground black pepper
(coarse-cracked pepper will do, if you don't
have a pepper mill.)

—

Yield: 6 servings, each with 1 gram of
carbohydrates, a trace of fiber, and 1 gram
of protein.

Blend all the ingredients, and store in the refrigerator, in a container with a tight-fitting lid.

Creamy Garlic Dressing

Look at all that garlic! If you plan to get kissed, make sure you share this salad with the object of your affections.

½ cup mayonnaise

Pinch each of pepper and salt

8 cloves garlic, crushed

2 tablespoons olive oil

2 tablespoons wine vinegar

—

Yield: 6 servings, each with 2 grams of
carbohydrates, a trace of fiber, and a trace
of protein.

Combine all the ingredients well, and store in the refrigerator, in a container with a tight-fitting lid.

> **NOTE**
>
> This is only enough for one big salad, but I wouldn't double it; I'd make this one fresh so the garlic flavor will be better.

Caesar Dressing

4 tablespoons lemon juice

¼ cup olive oil

1 teaspoon pepper

1½ teaspoons Worcestershire sauce

1 clove garlic, peeled and smashed

½ teaspoon salt or Vege-Sal

1 raw egg

½ cup grated Parmesan

2 inches anchovy paste (you could use an anchovy fillet or two if you prefer, but anchovy paste is handier, and it keeps forever in the fridge)

—

Yield: 8 servings, each with 1 gram of carbohydrates, a trace of fiber, and 3 grams of protein.

Put everything in a blender, run it for a minute, and toss with one really huge Caesar salad—dinner-party-sized—or a couple of smaller ones. Use it up pretty quickly, and keep it refrigerated because of the raw egg.

NOTE

If you'd like this a little thicker, you could add ¼ teaspoon of guar or xanthan to the mix.

Coleslaw Dressing

Virtually all commercial coleslaw dressing is simply full of sugar, which is a shame, since cabbage is a very low-carb vegetable. I just love coleslaw, so I came up with a sugar-free dressing.

½ cup mayonnaise

½ cup sour cream

1 to 1½ tablespoons apple cider vinegar

1 to 1½ teaspoons prepared mustard

½ to 1 teaspoon salt or Vege-Sal

½ to 1 packet artificial sweetener, or 1 teaspoon of Splenda

—

Yield: 12 servings, each with 1 gram of carbohydrates, with a trace of fiber, and a trace of protein.

Combine all the ingredients well, and toss with coleslaw. (See the recipes on page 104.)

NOTE

You may, of course, vary these proportions to taste. Also, a teaspoon or so of celery seed can be nice in this, for a little variety. I use this much dressing for a whole head of cabbage. If you're used to commercial coleslaw, which tends to be simply swimming in dressing, you may want to double this, or use this recipe for half a head.

CHAPTER 9

Condiments, Seasonings, and Sauces

Once you start reading labels, you'll be shocked at how many of your favorite seasonings, sauces, and especially condiments are simply loaded with sugar, corn syrup, cornstarch, flour, and other things you'd rather keep to a minimum. Most brands of ketchup have 4 grams of carbohydrates per tablespoon (15 g), for heaven's sake, and barbecue sauce tends to run even higher! You can carve significant chunks of carbohydrates out of your diet by making your own sauces at home, instead.

Stir-Fry Sauce

If you like Chinese food, make this up and keep it on hand. Then you can just throw any sort of meat and vegetables in your wok or skillet and have a meal in minutes.

½ cup soy sauce

½ cup dry sherry

2 cloves garlic, crushed

2 tablespoons grated fresh ginger

2 teaspoons Splenda

Combine the ingredients in a container with a tight-fitting lid, and refrigerate until you're ready to use.

—
Yield: 1 cup. Each 2-tablespoon serving has 2 grams of carbohydrates, no fiber, and no protein.

Not-Very-Authentic Peanut Sauce

This is inauthentic because I used substitutes for such traditional ingredients as lemon grass and fish sauce. I wanted a recipe that tasted good but could be made without a trip to specialty grocery store.

1 piece of fresh ginger about the size of a walnut, peeled and thinly sliced across the grain

½ cup natural peanut butter, creamy

½ cup chicken broth

1½ teaspoons lemon juice

1½ teaspoons soy sauce

¼ teaspoon Tabasco sauce

1 large or 2 small cloves garlic, crushed

1½ teaspoons Splenda

Put all the ingredients in a blender, and run it until everything is well combined and smooth. If you'd like it a little thinner, add another tablespoon of chicken broth.

—
Yield: about 2 cups, or 16 servings, each with 2 grams of carbohydrates, a trace of fiber, and 2 grams of protein.

Hoisin Sauce

This Chinese sauce is usually made from fermented soybean paste, which has tons of sugar in it. Peanut butter is inauthentic, but it tastes quite good here.

4 tablespoons soy sauce

2 tablespoons creamy natural peanut butter

2 tablespoons Splenda

2 teaspoons white vinegar

1 clove garlic, crushed

2 teaspoons toasted sesame oil

⅛ teaspoon Chinese Five Spice powder

Put all the ingredients in a blender, and run it until everything is smooth and well combined. Store in a snap-top container.

—

Yield: roughly ⅓ cup. Each 1-tablespoon serving contains 2 grams of carbohy-drates, a trace of fiber, and 2 grams of protein.

Hollandaise for Sissies

4 egg yolks

1 cup sour cream

1 tablespoon lemon juice

½ teaspoon salt or Vege-Sal

Dash of Tabasco

Put all the ingredients in a heavy-bottomed saucepan or the top of a double boiler. Whisk everything together well, let it heat through, and serve it over vegetables.

—

Yield: 6 to 8 servings, each with about 2 grams of carbohydrates, a trace of fiber, and 3 grams of protein.

> **NOTE**
>
> You'll need either a double boiler or a heat diffuser for this; it needs very gentle heat. If you're using a double boiler, you want the water in the bottom hot, but not boiling.

Taco Seasoning

Many store-bought seasoning blends include sugar or cornstarch—my food counter book says that several popular brands have 5 grams of carbs in 2 teaspoons! This is low-carb, very easy to put together, tastes great, and is even cheaper than the premixed stuff.

2 tablespoons chili powder

1½ tablespoons cumin

1½ tablespoons paprika

1 tablespoon onion powder

1 tablespoon garlic powder

⅛ to ¼ teaspoon cayenne pepper
(less makes a more mild seasoning,
more takes the spice up a notch)

—

Yield: about 8 tablespoons, or 4 batches worth. 2 tablespoons will add just under 2 grams of carbohydrates to a 4-ounce serving of taco meat.

Combine all the ingredients, blending well, and store in an airtight container. Use 2 tablespoons of this mixture to flavor 1 pound of ground beef, turkey, or chicken.

Chicken Seasoning

This is wonderful sprinkled over chicken before roasting.

3 tablespoons salt

1 teaspoon paprika

1 teaspoon onion powder

1 teaspoon garlic powder

1 teaspoon curry powder

½ teaspoon black pepper

—

Yield: just over ¼ cup. There are 7 grams of carb in this whole recipe and 1 gram of fiber, for a total of 6 grams of usable carbs, so the amount in the teaspoon or so you sprinkle over a piece of chicken is negligible.

Combine all the ingredients well, and store in a salt shaker or the shaker from an old container of herbs. Sprinkle over chicken before roasting; I use it to season at the table, as well.

Cajun Seasoning

This New Orleans–style seasoning is good sprinkled over chicken, steak, pork, fish, or just about anything else you care to try it on.

2½ tablespoons paprika

2 tablespoons salt

2 tablespoons garlic powder

1 tablespoon black pepper

1 tablespoon onion powder

1 tablespoon cayenne pepper

1 tablespoon dried oregano

1 tablespoon dried thyme

Combine all ingredients thoroughly, and store in an airtight container.

—

Yield: ⅔ cup. In the entire batch there are 37 grams of carbohydrates and 9 grams of fiber, for a total of 28 grams of usable carbs. Considering how spicy this is, you're unlikely to use more than a teaspoon or two at a time, and 1 teaspoon has just 1 gram of carbohydrates and a trace of fiber.

Jerk Seasoning

Sprinkle this over chicken, pork chops, or fish before cooking for an instant hit of hot, sweet, and spicy flavor.

1 tablespoon onion flakes

2 teaspoons ground thyme

1 teaspoon ground allspice

¼ teaspoon ground cinnamon

1 teaspoon black pepper

1 teaspoon cayenne pepper

1 tablespoon onion powder

2 teaspoons salt

¼ teaspoon ground nutmeg

2 tablespoons Splenda

Combine all the ingredients, and store in an airtight container.

—

Yield: about ⅓ cup. Each teaspoon contains 1 gram of carbohydrates, a trace of fiber, and no protein.

Dana's No-Sugar Ketchup

Store-bought ketchup has more sugar in it per ounce than ice cream does! This great-tasting ketchup has all the flavor of your favorite brand, without the high carb count. The guar or xanthan isn't essential, but it makes your ketchup a little thicker and helps keep the water from separating out if you don't use it up quickly.

1 can (6 ounces) tomato paste

⅔ cup cider vinegar

⅓ cup water

⅓ cup Splenda

2 tablespoons finely minced onion

2 cloves garlic, crushed

1 teaspoon salt or Vege-Sal

⅛ teaspoon ground allspice

⅛ teaspoon ground cloves

⅛ teaspoon pepper

¼ teaspoon guar or xanthan

—
Yield: 1½ cups of ketchup. 1 tablespoon has 2.25 grams of carbohydrates, a trace of fiber, and a trace of protein.

Put all the ingredients in a blender, and run the blender until the bits of onion disappear. (You'll have to scrape down the sides as you go, because this mixture is thick.) Store in the refrigerator, in a container with a tight-fitting lid.

Low-Carb Steak Sauce

¼ cup Dana's No-Sugar Ketchup (see above)

1 tablespoon Worcestershire sauce

1 teaspoon lemon juice

—
Yield: 5 servings of 1 tablespoon, each with 2.25 grams of carbohydrates, a trace of fiber, and a trace of protein.

Combine well and store in an airtight container in the fridge.

Cocktail Sauce

Use this for dipping your cold, boiled shrimp in, of course. Commercial cocktail sauce, like so many other condiments, is full of sugar.

¼ cup Dana's No-Sugar Ketchup (see page 119)

1 teaspoon prepared horseradish

2 or 3 drops Tabasco

½ teaspoon lemon juice

Just stir together, and dip!

—

Yield: ¼ cup, with 10 grams of carbohydrate, a trace of fiber, and a trace of protein in the whole batch.

Aioli

This is basically just very garlicky mayonnaise. It's good on all kinds of vegetables, and on fish, too.

4 cloves garlic, crushed very thoroughly

1 egg

¼ teaspoon salt

2 tablespoons lemon juice

½ to ⅔ cup olive oil

Put the garlic, egg, salt, and lemon juice in a blender. Run the blender for a second, and then pour in the oil in a very thin stream, as you would when making mayonnaise. Turn off the blender when the sauce is thickened.

—

Yield: about 1 cup, or 8 servings of 2 tablespoons, each with 1 gram of carbohydrates, only a trace of fiber, and 1 gram of protein.

Tequila Lime Marinade

⅓ cup lime juice (bottled is fine)

⅓ cup water

3 tablespoons tequila

1 tablespoon Splenda

1 tablespoon soy sauce

2 cloves garlic, crushed.

—

Yield: roughly ¾ cup (enough for a dozen boneless, skinless chicken breasts or a couple of pounds of shrimp). In the whole batch there are 13 grams of carbohydrates and 1 gram of fiber, for a total of 12 grams of usable carbs and no protein, but since you drain most of the marinade off, you won't get more than a gram or two of carbs total.

Combine the ingredients, and store in the refrigerator until ready to use.

Teriyaki Sauce

Good on chicken, beef, fish—just about anything.

½ cup soy sauce

¼ cup dry sherry

1 clove garlic, crushed

2 tablespoons Splenda

1 tablespoon grated fresh ginger

—

Yield: just over ¾ cup. Each 1-tablespoon serving will have about 3 grams of carbohydrates, a trace of fiber, and a trace of protein.

Combine all the ingredients, and refrigerate until ready to use.

Jerk Marinade

Jerk is a Jamaican way of life. Make it with one pepper if you want it just nicely hot or with two peppers if you want it traditional—also known as take-the-top-of-your-head-off hot.

1 or 2 Scotch Bonnet or habenero peppers, with or without seeds (the seeds are the hottest part)

½ small onion

3 tablespoons oil

1 tablespoon ground allspice

2 tablespoons grated fresh ginger

1 tablespoon soy sauce

1 teaspoon dried thyme

1 bay leaf, crumbled

¼ teaspoon cinnamon

1 tablespoon Splenda

2 cloves garlic, crushed

—
Yield: enough for about 4 servings of meat, each serving serving of Jerk Marinade adding 4 grams of carbohydrates and 1 gram of fiber, for a total of 3 grams of usable carbs and no protein.

Put all the ingredients in a food processor with the S blade in place, and process until it's fairly smooth. (You'll get a soft paste that looks like mud but smells like heaven!) Smear this over the meat of your choice, and let it sit for a day before cooking. Always wash your hands after handling hot peppers!

> **NOTE**
>
> If you just can't take the heat, you can chicken out and use a jalapeño or two instead of the habeneros or Scotch Bonnets, and your jerk marinade will be quite mild, as these things go. But remember: There is no such thing as a truly mild jerk sauce.

Looing Sauce

This is a Chinese sauce for "red cooking." You stew things in it, and it imparts a wonderful flavor to just about any sort of meat.

2 cups soy sauce

1 star anise

½ cup dry sherry (the cheap stuff is fine)

4 tablespoons Splenda

1 tablespoon grated fresh ginger

4 cups water

—
Yield: 6½ cups of looing sauce, or plenty to submerge your food in. In the whole batch there are about 50 grams of usable carbohydrates, but only a very small amount of that is transferred to the foods you stew in it.

Combine the ingredients well and use the mixture to stew things in. (Specifically, see Looed Pork on page 96.) After using Looing Sauce, you can strain it and refrigerate or freeze it to use again, if you like.

> **NOTE**
>
> Star anise is available in Asian markets, and my health food store carries it, too. It actually does look like a star, and it's essential to the recipe. Don't try to substitute regular anise.

Cranberry Sauce

Unbelievably easy, and good with roast chicken or turkey—as though you needed to be told!

½ teaspoon plain gelatin (optional)

1 cup water

1 bag (12 ounces) fresh cranberries

1 cup Splenda

—
Yield: roughly 2 cups. Each 2-tablespoon serving will have 4 grams of carbohydrates and 1 gram of fiber, for a total of 3 grams of usable carbs.

Combine water, cranberries, and Splenda in a sauce pan over medium-high heat. (If you're using the gelatin, dissolve it in ½ cup of the water, then add it to the cranberries and Splenda in a saucepan over medium-high heat.) Bring the mixture to a boil, and boil it hard until the cranberries pop. Keep it in a tightly covered jar in the fridge.

Cranberry Chutney

1 bag (12 ounces) cranberries

1 cup water

½ cup Splenda

2 cloves garlic, crushed

1 tablespoon pumpkin pie spice

⅛ teaspoon salt

—

Yield: roughly 2 cups. Each 2-tablespoon serving will have just over 3 grams of carbohydrates and 1 gram of fiber, for a total of 2 grams of usable carbs and only a trace of protein.

Combine all the ingredients in a saucepan over medium heat, bring it to a boil, and boil until the cranberries pop (7 to 8 minutes).

NOTE

This recipe improves if you let the boiled mixture sit for a while before serving. Try it with a little cinnamon, too.

Tootsie's Pesto

2 cups fresh basil leaves, washed and patted dry

4 good-size garlic cloves

1 cup shelled walnuts or pine nuts

1 cup extra-virgin olive oil

1 cup freshly grated Parmesan cheese

¼ cup freshly grated Romano cheese

Salt and pepper to taste

—

Yield: 2 cups. Each 1-tablespoon serving will have 1 gram of carbohydrates, a trace of fiber, and 2 grams of protein.

Combine the basil, garlic, and nuts, and chop in a food processor with the S blade. Leave the motor running, and add the olive oil in a slow steady stream.

Shut off the food processor, and add the Parmesan, Romano, a big pinch of salt, and a liberal grinding of pepper. Process briefly to blend.

Green Tomato Chutney

4 quarts green tomatoes, cut into chunks

3 cups apple cider vinegar

1 whole ginger root, sliced into very thin rounds

5 or 6 cloves garlic, thinly sliced

1 tablespoon whole cloves

5 or 6 sticks whole cinnamon

½ cup Splenda

1 tablespoon blackstrap molasses

3 teaspoons stevia/FOS blend

—
Yield: roughly 2 quarts. Each 2-tablespoon serving will have 5 grams of carbohydrates and 1 gram of fiber, for a total of 4 grams of usable carbs and no protein.

Combine all the ingredients in a large stainless steel or enamel kettle—no iron, no aluminum. (This is an acidic mixture, and if you use iron or aluminum you'll end up with your chutney chock full of iron, which will turn it blackish, or aluminum, which simply isn't good for you.) Simmer on low for 3 to 4 hours. Store in tightly closed containers in the refrigerator.

Duck Sauce

1 bag (1 pound) unsweetened frozen peaches or 2½ to 3 cups sliced, peeled fresh peaches

½ cup water

2 tablespoons cider vinegar

2 tablespoon Splenda

¼ teaspoon blackstrap molasses

⅛ teaspoon salt

1 teaspoon soy sauce

1 clove garlic, crushed

—
Yield: about 2 cups. Each 2-tablespoon serving has 3 grams of carbohydrates and 1 gram of fiber, for a total of 2 grams of usable carbs and no protein.

Put all the ingredients in a heavy-bottomed saucepan, and bring them to a simmer. Cook, uncovered, until the peaches are soft (about 30 minutes).

Puree the duck sauce in a blender, if you like, or do what I do: simply mash the sauce with a potato masher or a fork. (I like the texture better this way.)

CHAPTER 10

Sweet Desserts

I am of two minds about this chapter (a chapter which, by the way, contains recipes for treats as delicious as any sugary desserts you've ever made). On the one hand, I think it's a bad idea to get in the habit of eating these sugarless sweets with the same frequency with which you used to eat the sugary stuff. I feel strongly that weaning yourself away from wanting sweets all the time, from not considering a meal complete until you've had a dessert, is a very good and important thing.

Mom's Chocolate Chip Cookies

With this recipe, I assume the title of Low-Carb Cookie God.

1 cup butter, at room temperature

1 ½ cups Splenda

1½ teaspoons blackstrap molasses

2 eggs

1 cup ground almonds

1 cup vanilla-flavored whey protein powder

¼ cup oat bran

1 teaspoon baking soda

1 teaspoon salt

1 cup chopped walnuts or pecans

12 ounces sugar-free chocolate chips

—
Yield: about 4½ dozen cookies,
each with 3 grams of carbohydrates, a trace of fiber, and 5 grams of protein. (This carbohydrate count does not include the polyols used to sweeten the sugar-free chocolate, since it remains largely undigested and unabsorbed.)

Preheat the oven to 375°F.

Use an electric mixer to beat the butter, Splenda, and molasses until creamy and well blended. Add the eggs, one at a time, and beat well after each addition.

In a separate bowl, stir together the ground almonds, protein powder, oat bran, baking soda, and salt. Add this mixture, about ½ cup at a time, to the Splenda mixture, beating well after each ½-cup addition, until it's all beaten in. Stir in the nuts and chocolate chips.

Spray a cookie sheet with nonstick cooking spray, and drop the dough by rounded tablespoons onto it. These cookies will not spread and flatten as much as standard chocolate chip cookies, so if you want them flat, flatten them a bit now.

Bake for 10 minutes, or until golden. Cool on baking sheets for a couple minutes, then remove to wire racks to cool completely.

NOTES

• If you haven't ground your almonds yet, now would be a good time to do that, as well.

• If you can't get sugar-free chocolate chips, you need to make some from sugar-free chocolate bars. Break 7 or 8 of the bars, which are 1.3 to 1.5 ounces each, into three or four pieces each, and place the pieces in a food processor with the S blade in place. Pulse the food processor until your chocolate bars are in pieces about the same size as commercial chocolate morsels, and set them aside until you're ready to use them.

Peanut Butter Brownies

This was the first recipe I ever tried from *Diana Lee's Baking Low Carb*, and I've been recommending her book ever since. The peanut butter topping sinks to the bottom, and you get fudgy brownie on top and chewy peanut butter cookie on the bottom.

BROWNIE LAYER

5 tablespoons butter

¼ cup unsweetened baking cocoa

2 eggs

¼ cup heavy cream

¼ cup water

1 teaspoon vanilla extract

¼ cup Splenda

1 teaspoon liquid saccharine

¾ cup vanilla-flavored whey protein powder

2 tablespoons oat flour

1 tablespoon baking powder

PEANUT BUTTER TOPPING

¼ cup natural peanut butter

3 tablespoons butter

2 tablespoons Splenda

1 egg

2 tablespoons vanilla-flavored whey protein powder

—

Yield: 16 brownies, each with 5 grams of carbohydrates and 1 gram of fiber, for a total of 4 grams of usable carbs and 12 grams of protein.

Preheat the oven to 350°F.

Melt the butter and stir in the cocoa. Add the eggs, cream, water, vanilla, Splenda, and saccharine, and mix well.

Add the protein powder, oat flour, and baking powder, and mix just until well moistened.

Spray an 8 x 8-inch baking pan with nonstick cooking spray, and pour the batter into it.

Mix the peanut butter, butter, Splenda, egg, and protein powder together, and spoon the mixture on top of the brownie batter. Bake for 15 minutes—do not overbake.

Hazelnut Crust

This is a great substitute for a graham cracker crumb crust with any cheesecake. And I think it tastes even better than the original.

1½ cups hazelnuts

⅓ cup vanilla-flavored whey protein powder

4 tablespoons butter, melted

—

Yield: assuming 12 slices of cheesecake, this crust will add to each slice 4 grams of carbohydrates and 1 gram of fiber, for a total of 3 grams of usable carbs and 10 grams of protein.

Preheat the oven to 350°F.

Put the hazelnuts in a food processor with the S blade in place. Pulse the processor until the hazelnuts are ground to a medium-fine texture. Add the protein powder and butter, and pulse to combine.

Spray the pie plate or springform pan, depending on which your recipe specifies, with nonstick cooking spray, and press this mixture firmly and evenly into the pan. Don't try to build your crust too high up the sides, but if you're using a springform pan, be sure to cover the seam around the bottom and press the crust into place firmly over it.

Place your crust in a preheated oven on the bottom rack, and bake for 12 to 15 minutes, or until lightly browned and slightly pulling away from the sides of the pan. Remove the crust from the oven, and let it cool while you make the filling.

ALMOND CRUST. Here's another great nut crust for you to try. Just substitute 1½ cups almonds for the hazelnuts in the **HAZELNUT CRUST** (above) and decrease the vanilla-flavored whey protein powder to ¼ cup. Follow the directions to make the crust, and bake for 10 to 12 minutes, or until lightly golden. Cool.

—

Yield: assuming 12 slices of cheesecake, this crust will add to each slice 4 grams of carbohydrates and 2 grams of fiber, for a total of 2 grams of usable carbs and 7 grams of protein.

Cheesecake to Go with Fruit

This lemon-vanilla cheesecake is wonderful with strawberries, blueberries, cherries—any fruit you care to use. It also makes a nice breakfast.

2 cups cottage cheese

2 eggs

½ cup sour cream

¼ cup vanilla-flavored whey protein powder

¼ cup Splenda

Grated rind and juice of 1 fresh lemon

1 teaspoon vanilla extract

1 Hazelnut Crust or Almond Crust
(see page 129), prebaked in a large,
deep pie plate

—

Yield: 12 servings, each with 8 grams of carbohydrates and 2 grams of fiber, for a total of 6 grams of usable carbs and 21 grams of protein. (Analysis includes crust.)

Preheat the oven to 375°F.

Put the cottage cheese, eggs, sour cream, protein powder, Splenda, lemon rind and juice, and vanilla extract in a blender, and blend until very smooth.

Pour into the prebaked crust. Place the cake on the top rack of the oven, and place a flat pan of water on the bottom rack. Bake for 30 to 40 minutes. Cool, then chill well before serving.

NOTE

Serve this cheesecake with the fruit of your choice. I like to serve it with thawed frozen, unsweetened strawberries, blueberries, or peaches, mashed coarsely with a fork and sweetened slightly with Splenda. If you use 1½ cups of strawberries with 2 tablespoons Splenda for the whole cake, you'll add 2 grams of carbohydrates per slice, plus a trace of fiber and a trace of protein. Use 1½ cups sour cherries—you can get these canned, with no added sugar—and sweeten them with ¼ cup Splenda, and you'll add 3 grams per slice. I'm lucky enough to have a sour cherry tree, and cherry cheesecake is one of the joys of early summer around here!

Sunshine Cheesecake

This has a lovely, creamy texture and a bright, sunshiney orange flavor. Using the stevia/FOS blend keeps the carb count very low.

1 cup cottage cheese

1 package (8 ounces) cream cheese, softened

1 cup sour cream

4 eggs

Grated rind of 1 orange

1 tablespoon orange extract

1 tablespoon plus 1 teaspoon stevia/FOS blend

2 tablespoons lemon juice

Tiny pinch salt

1 Hazelnut Crust or Almond Crust (see page 129), prebaked in a springform pan

—
Yield: 12 servings, each with 8 grams of carbohydrates and 2 grams of fiber, for a total of 6 grams of usable carbs and 17 grams of protein. (Analysis includes crust.)

Put the cottage cheese, cream cheese, sour cream, eggs, orange rind, orange extract, stevia, lemon juice, and salt in a blender, and run the blender until everything is well-blended and a bit fluffy.

Pour into the prebaked crust. Place the cake on the top rack of the oven, and place a flat pan of water on the bottom rack. Bake for 50 minutes. The cheesecake will still jiggle slightly in the center when you take it out.

Cool, then chill well before serving.

NOTE

This is wonderful with sugar-free chocolate syrup. Many grocery stores carry it; it's worth your while to take a look-see.

Great Balls of Protein!

You may recognize this updated version of an old health food standby.

1 jar (16 ounces) natural peanut butter, oil and all

2 cups vanilla-flavored whey protein powder

Splenda, saccharine, stevia, or whatever sweetener you prefer (optional)

Sesame seeds (optional)

Unsweetened shredded coconut (optional)

Sugar-free chocolate bars (optional)

Unsweetened cocoa powder (optional)

Splenda (optional)

—
Yield: About 50 balls, each with 3 grams of carbohydrates, a trace of fiber, and 10 grams of protein. (Analysis does not include coatings for balls.)

NOTES

• This is easiest to make if you have a powerful stand mixer or a heavy-duty food processor. If you don't, don't try to use a smaller appliance—you'll only burn it out and destroy it! Rather than dooming your old mixer, just roll up your sleeves, scrub your hands, and dive in.

• If you're using stevia, dissolve it in a couple of tablespoons of water and sprinkle it evenly over the mixture before working it in, or it's not likely to spread throughout the mixture very well. Actually, it's best to sprinkle any sweetener evenly before combining it with a mixture this thick.

Thoroughly combine the peanut butter with the protein powder. (I find that working in about ⅓ cup of the protein powder at a time is about right.) This should make a stiff, somewhat crumbly dough.

Work the sweetener of your choice (if using) into the dough. My whey protein powder is sweetened with stevia, and I find that that's enough sweetener for me. But if you want your Great Balls of Protein to be sweeter, simply add sweetener.

Roll into balls about 1 inch in diameter.

It's nice to coat these with something. If you like sesame seeds, you can toast them by shaking them in a dry, heavy skillet over medium heat until they start popping and jumping around the pan, and then roll the balls in them while they're still warm. You could roll them in coconut, if you prefer; most health food stores carry it unsweetened and shredded. Again, you can toast it lightly in a dry frying pan, and add a little Splenda. Or you could melt sugar-free chocolate bars, and dip your Balls of Protein in chocolate—although it would probably be simpler to chop them up and mix them in. Another option is to roll them in unsweetened cocoa mixed with a little Splenda.

Whipped Topping

The pudding adds a very nice texture to this topping, and it helps the whipped cream "stand up," as well as adding a slightly sweet vanilla flavor to the cream, of course.

1 cup heavy cream, well chilled

1 tablespoon vanilla sugar-free instant pudding powder

—
Yield: About 2 cups, or 16 servings of 2 tablespoons, each with only a trace of carbohydrates, no fiber, and a trace of protein.

Whip the cream and pudding mix together until the cream is stiff.

Strawberry Sauce

Traditionally, Couer a la Crème is served with fresh strawberries, but I make this for Valentine's Day, and I'm generally not impressed with the quality of the fresh strawberries I can get in February. I'd rather use frozen.

1 bag (1 pound) frozen, unsweetened strawberries, thawed

1 tablespoon lemon juice

2 or 3 tablespoons Splenda

—
Yield: 8 servings, each with 6 grams of carbohydrates and 1 gram of fiber, for a total of 5 grams of usable carbs and only a trace of protein.

Simply pour your strawberries and any liquid in the package into a bowl, and stir in the lemon juice and Splenda. Mash your strawberries a little with a fork, if you'd like; I like mine fairly chunky.

Helen's Chocolate Bread Pudding

Helen was my dad's mom, and this was our family's traditional Christmas dessert the whole time I was growing up. People have threatened to marry into the family to get the secret recipe, but since this is the decarbed version, it's not secret! It is still high-carb enough that you'll want to save it for a special occasion, though.

2 cups half-and-half

1 cup heavy cream

1 cup water

6 slices "lite" white bread (5 grams of usable carbs per slice or less—the squishiest you can find)

3 ounces unsweetened baking chocolate

⅔ cup Splenda

2 eggs, beaten

1 teaspoon vanilla extract

Pinch salt

—

Yield: 8 servings, each with 12 grams of carbohydrates and just over 1 gram of fiber, for a total of 11 grams of usable carbs and 7 grams of protein.

Preheat the oven to 375°F.

Combine the half-and-half, cream, and water, and scald; bring it just up to a simmer.

While it's heating, spray a large casserole with nonstick cooking spray, tear the bread into small bits, and put them in the dish. Pour the hot half-and-half mixture over the bread, and let it sit for 10 minutes.

Melt the chocolate, and add it to the bread mixture; it's good to use a little of the hot cream to rinse out the pan you melted the chocolate in, so you get all of it. Stir well. Now stir in the Splenda, eggs, vanilla, and salt, mixing very well. Bake for 1 hour, or until firm. Serve with Not-So-Hard Sauce (see opposite).

Not-So-Hard Sauce

Traditional hard sauce is made with sugar, butter, and egg, plus vanilla, rum, or brandy, and when it's refrigerated it gets quite hard—hence the name. However, with Splenda instead of sugar, my hard sauce just didn't work—it fell apart in little globs. I added cream cheese, and it all came together, but it doesn't get quite so hard when refrigerated, which is why this is Not-So-Hard Sauce. It still tastes great, though!

1 cup Splenda

5 tablespoons butter, softened

⅛ teaspoon salt

1 teaspoon vanilla extract

1 egg

1 ounce cream cheese, softened

Nutmeg

—

Yield: About 1 cup, or a 2-tablespoons serving of sauce for each serving of Helen's Chocolate Bread Pudding (see page 455). Each serving will have 3 grams of carbohydrates, no fiber, and 1 gram of protein.

Use an electric mixer to beat the Splenda and butter together until well blended. Beat in the salt, vanilla extract, and egg. At this point, you'll be sure you've made a dreadful mistake.

Beat in the cream cheese, and watch the sauce smooth out! Mix very well, until light and fluffy. Pile your Not-So-Hard Sauce into a pretty serving dish, sprinkle it lightly with nutmeg, and refrigerate until well-chilled.

Zucchini-Carrot Cake

About 1¼ cups hazelnuts

2 eggs

½ cup oil

⅔ cup Splenda

½ cup yogurt

½ cup vanilla-flavored whey protein powder

1 teaspoon baking soda

½ teaspoon salt

1½ teaspoons cinnamon

¼ teaspoon nutmeg

¾ cup shredded zucchini

¼ cup shredded carrot

—

Yield: 8 generous servings, each with 8 grams of carbohydrates and 2 grams of fiber, for a total of 6 grams of usable carbs and 16 grams of protein.

Preheat the oven to 350°F.

In a food processor with the S blade in place, use the pulse control to grind the hazelnuts to a mealy consistency. (You want 1 ½ cups of ground hazelnuts when you're done, and for some inexplicable reason they seem to actually grow a little rather than shrink a little when you grind them.) Set the ground hazelnuts aside.

In a large mixing bowl, whisk the eggs until well blended. Add the oil, yogurt, ground hazelnuts, protein powder, baking soda, Splenda, salt, cinnamon, and nutmeg, mixing well after each addition. (It's especially important that the baking soda be well distributed through the mixture.) Add the zucchini and carrots last, mixing well.

Thoroughly coat a ring mold or bundt pan with nonstick cooking spray, and turn the batter into it.

If you sprayed your pan ahead of time, give it another shot just before adding the batter. And don't expect the batter to fill the pan to the rim; it fills my bundt pan about halfway.

Bake for 45 minutes and turn out gently onto a wire rack to cool.

NOTE

This doesn't need a darned thing—it's simply delicious exactly the way it is. If you wish to gild the lily, however, you could top it with whipped topping, pumpkin cream, or cream cheese frosting. This cake, by the way, makes a fabulous breakfast, and since it's loaded with protein and good fats, it should keep you going all morning.

Gingerbread

I've always loved gingerbread, and this is as good as any high-carb gingerbread I've ever had! Don't worry about that zucchini; it completely disappears, leaving only moistness behind.

1 cup ground almonds (or ⅔ cup raw almonds finely ground in a food processor)

½ cup vanilla-flavored whey protein powder

1 teaspoon baking soda

½ teaspoon salt

2½ teaspoons ground ginger

½ teaspoon ground cinnamon

½ cup Splenda

½ cup plain yogurt

¼ cup oil

1 teaspoon blackstrap molasses

1 egg

2 tablespoons water

½ cup shredded zucchini

—

Yield: 9 servings, each with 9 grams of carbohydrates, a trace of fiber, and 17 grams of protein.

Preheat the oven to 350°F.

In a mixing bowl, combine the almonds, protein powder, baking soda, salt, ginger, cinnamon, and Splenda, and mix them well.

In a separate bowl or measuring cup, whisk together the yogurt, oil, molasses, egg, and water. Pour into the dry ingredients, and whisk until everything is well combined and there are no dry spots. Add the zucchini, and whisk briefly to distribute evenly.

Spray an 8 x 8-inch baking pan with nonstick cooking spray, and turn the batter into it. Bake for 30 minutes, or until a toothpick inserted in the middle comes out clean.

NOTE

Try serving this with Whipped Topping (see page 133).

Strawberries in Wine

Simple, and simply delicious.

8 ounces fresh strawberries

½ cup burgundy wine

1 tablespoon Splenda

Cinnamon stick

—
Yield: 4 servings, each with 8 grams of carbohydrates and 3 grams of fiber, for a total of 5 grams of usable carbs and 1 gram of protein.

Hull the strawberries, and slice or cut them into quarters.

Mix the wine and the Splenda, and pour the mixture over the berries. Add the cinnamon stick and refrigerate, stirring from time to time, for at least 12 hours (but 2 days wouldn't hurt!).

Mockahlua

My sister, a longtime Kahlua fan, says this is addictive. And my husband demanded to know, "How did you do that?" You can make this with decaf if caffeine bothers you.

2½ cups water

3 cups Splenda

3 tablespoons instant coffee crystals

1 teaspoon vanilla

1 bottle (750 milliliters) 100-proof vodka (use the cheap stuff)

—

Yield: 32 servings of 1½ ounces—a standard "shot." Each will have 2 grams of carbohydrates, no fiber, and the merest trace of protein.

In a large pitcher or measuring cup, combine the water, Splenda, coffee crystals, and vanilla. Stir until the coffee and Splenda are completely dissolved.

Pour the mixture through a funnel into a 1.5- or 2-liter bottle. (A clean 1.5-liter wine bottle works fine, so long as you've saved the cork.) Pour in the vodka. Cork, and shake well.

MOCHAHLUA. Try this one if you like a little chocolate with your coffee. Just cut the water back to 1½ cups and substitute a 12-ounce bottle of sugar-free chocolate coffee flavoring syrup for the Splenda and vanilla. This has only a trace of carbohydrates per shot, because the liquid Splenda used to sweeten the chocolate coffee flavoring syrup doesn't have the maltodextrin used to bulk the granular Splenda.

MOCKAHLUA AND CREAM. This makes a nice "little something" to serve at the end of a dinner party, in lieu of a heavier dessert. For each serving you'll need a shot of Mockahlua (or Mochalua) and 2 shots of heavy cream. Simply mix and sip!

—

Yield: Each Serving has 4 grams of carbohydrates, no fiber, and 2 grams of protein.

A Refresher on Measurements

Just in case these details have slipped your mind since junior high school home ec class:

3 teaspoons = 1 tablespoon

2 tablespoons = 1 fluid ounce

2 ounces = ¼ cup

4 ounces = ½ cup

8 ounces = 1 cup

2 cups = 1 pint

4 cups = 1 quart

2 pints = 1 quart

4 quarts = 1 gallon

Help! I Use the Metric System!

The problem with being an American cookbook author is that your recipes end up being confusing to the vast majority of the world—namely, the millions of folks out there who don't use quarts, cups, teaspoons, and tablespoons, and whose ovens are calibrated for Celsius rather than Fahrenheit. That most of the world measures dry ingredients by weight rather than volume just adds to the confusion.

Here, for all you nice folks who live in that great big world outside the United States, are some useful measurement conversions. I'm afraid I can't convert measurements of volume to measurements of weight, but I can give you the volumes in liters and the oven temperatures in Celsius. It's good to know that a liter and a quart are so close as to make almost no difference and that for our purposes, we're going to assume they're the same. Be aware that there are two different sorts of ounces in the measurement system used in America—an ounce of weight, and a "fluid ounce," which is measure of volume equal to 2 tablespoons. If a liquid is being measured in ounces, this will always refer to a fluid ounce, rather than an ounce of weight.

Measurements of Volume

1 quart = 1 liter

1 cup = 250 milliliters

¾ cup = 200 milliliters`

½ cup = 125 milliliters`

⅓ cup = 105 milliliters

¼ cup = 75 milliliters

1 fluid ounce = 30 milliliters

1 tablespoon = 15 milliliters

1 teaspoon = 5 milliliters

Measurements of Weight

1 ounce = 28.4 grams, but in most cases you can round to 25 or 30

1 pound = 454 grams, or about half a kilo

In America, we measure butter both by the pound and by volumetric measurements:

1 pound butter = 2 cups

1 stick butter = ¼ pound = ½ cup = 8 tablespoons = 113 grams

1 cup butter = 226 grams

1 tablespoon butter = 14 grams

Oven Temperatures

225°F = 110°C	375°F = 190°C
250°F = 130°C	400°F = 200°C
275°F = 140°C	425°F = 220°C
300°F = 150°C	450°F = 230°C
325°F = 170°C	475°F = 240°C
350°F = 180°C	

Index

Printed in the USA
CPSIA information can be obtained
at www.ICGtesting.com
LVHW072231010923
756670LV00002B/5